Ageless and Mindful Movement

Wall Pilates Practices for Every Age with Effective Exercises Tailored for All Fitness Levels

Clara Wells

of ConTents

in the rendering of legal, financial, medical or professional advice. The content within this book has been derived from various sources. Please consult a licensed professional before attempting any techniques outlined in this book.

By reading this document, the reader agrees that under no circumstances is the author responsible for any losses, direct or indirect, that are incurred as a result of the use of the information contained within this document, including, but not limited to, errors, omissions, or inaccuracies.

Introduction

Have you ever felt that your body is capable of more than it currently demonstrates? Imagine waking up each day with a sense of strength and flexibility, prepared to tackle whatever life throws your way—all through the gentle practice of Wall Pilates. This transformative exercise method holds the promise of revitalizing not only your physical well-being but also your mental clarity, offering a sanctuary of calm amid the hustle and bustle of daily life. Whether you are a senior looking to maintain functional strength or a beginner embarking on a fitness journey, Wall Pilates provides an accessible path toward enhanced health.

Wall Pilates is not just another fitness trend; it is a thoughtful, low-impact exercise technique designed to improve your overall quality of life. Utilizing the support and stability of a wall, this method emphasizes controlled movements that enhance muscle tone, flexibility, and balance. The unique aspect of Wall Pilates lies in its inclusivity—crafted to cater to diverse physical abilities, ensuring that everyone, regardless of age or experience level, can partake and benefit from it. The gentle nature of Wall Pilates makes it particularly beneficial for seniors seeking to stay active without risking injury, while beginners will appreciate the structured approach that builds confidence and encourages steady progress.

Wall Pilates offers holistic benefits that go beyond just physical fitness. Imagine feeling more connected to your body, aware of each movement and breath as you engage in mindful practices incorporated into your workout routine. This exercise method fosters a comprehensive approach to wellness, intertwining physical activity with mental rejuvenation.

Embarking on a new fitness routine can often come with barriers and concerns. Physical limitations, a sense of intimidation, or simply not knowing where to start can all be daunting aspects. These are valid considerations, and it's essential to acknowledge them openly. Many people might think that exercises like Pilates are reserved for younger, more agile individuals. Yet, Wall Pilates is designed to be adaptable, with modifications and gentle guidance that make it accessible to everyone. With its focus on gradual progression, you can embark on this journey feeling safe and supported, gradually building strength and confidence.

One of the most enriching aspects of diving into Wall Pilates is the sense of community it fosters. As you turn the pages of this book, visualize yourself becoming part of a welcoming group of practitioners who share similar goals and challenges. Engaging with others who are exploring Wall Pilates can provide motivation, accountability, and a shared passion for health that transcends individual efforts. This sense of belonging can be incredibly uplifting, transforming your personal fitness journey into a collaborative endeavor filled with encouragement and camaraderie.

The decision to incorporate Wall Pilates into your life marks the beginning of a journey towards improved well-being—a commitment to yourself and to the joys that come with embracing a healthier lifestyle. This book serves as your guide, offering clear instructions and tailored modifications that ensure the exercises meet your specific needs. Whether you're looking to maintain the strength and independence you've cultivated over the years, or you're eagerly stepping into the world of fitness with curiosity and determination, Wall Pilates stands as a supportive ally.

Consider the daily impact of engaging in Wall Pilates. For seniors, this could mean continued independence, the ability to perform everyday tasks with ease, and a reduction in joint pain and stiffness. It promotes better posture, balance, and coordination, which are crucial for preventing falls and enhancing the overall quality of life. For beginners, Wall Pilates serves as an introduction to a sustainable fitness routine, one that respects the body's need for slow, deliberate engagement rather than rushed, high-intensity workouts. The emphasis on mindful movement enhances body awareness and helps cultivate a deeper connection between mind and body, setting the stage for long-term fitness success.

Wall Pilates fits seamlessly into various lifestyles, making it a practical choice regardless of your schedule. The simplicity of needing just a wall means you can practice at home, in the office, or even outdoors, creating opportunities to integrate these exercises into your daily routine effortlessly. The adaptability of Wall Pilates ensures that you can remain consistent, finding moments throughout your day to invest in your physical and mental health without the stress of arranging gym visits or complicated equipment.

The journey that lies ahead is one of empowerment and transformation. Embracing Wall Pilates allows you to take control of your health, understanding that small, consistent efforts lead to significant changes over time. By committing to this practice, you are investing in a future where strength, flexibility, and balance become pillars of your daily existence. Each movement, supported by the stability of the wall, becomes a step toward a more vibrant, resilient you.

So, let this book be your companion as you embark on this inspiring journey. Within these pages, you'll find the knowledge, encouragement, and support needed to make Wall Pilates a cornerstone of your wellness routine. Together, we will explore the possibilities, overcome challenges, and celebrate the milestones that define your path to greater health. Welcome to a community of individuals dedicated to the pursuit of balanced, fulfilling lives through the gentle yet powerful practice of Wall Pilates.

Chapter 1
Introduction to Wall Pilates

Wall Pilates combines the foundational principles of traditional Pilates with the unique advantage of utilizing a wall for support and resistance. This chapter delves into the origins and guiding principles of Wall Pilates, offering insights into its historical context and evolution. Developed by Joseph H. Pilates in the early 20th century, this form of exercise has grown to accommodate various fitness levels and age groups, making it an accessible and effective workout option.

Origin and Principles of Wall Pilates

To truly appreciate Wall Pilates, it is helpful to understand its historical context and how it evolved as an effective workout for people from various fitness backgrounds.

Historical Background

Pilates, originally known as "Contrology," was developed by Joseph H. Pilates in the early 20th century. During World War I, Joseph Pilates created exercises to help rehabilitate injured soldiers. His method focused on core strength, flexibility, and overall body control.

Joseph Pilates believed that mental and physical health were interconnected. He emphasized the importance of breathing and concentration in each movement, which formed the foundation of his exercises. As his studio grew in popularity, he introduced methods to help not just dancers but also everyday people. He wanted his exercises to be accessible, making it clear that everyone could benefit from them. His sessions blended strength training with restorative movements, creating a holistic approach that appealed to many.

The methods developed by Pilates spread beyond the confines of his studio. In the 1960s, several of his students became instructors, taking their knowledge into fitness clubs and gyms across the country. They adapted his exercises to fit different settings, making Pilates more mainstream. This expansion introduced a wave of new practitioners who put their spin on the original techniques. Some emphasized strength, while others focused more on flexibility. Despite these variations, the core principles remained intact, ensuring that the essence of Pilates lived on (Lim & Hyun, 2021).

Over time, Pilates gained popularity and evolved into various forms, including Wall Pilates. This variation incorporates many of the original principles but adapts the exercises to be performed against a wall. This modification provides extra stability and resistance, making it accessible to individuals at different fitness levels, particularly seniors and beginners.

Core Principles

The core principles of Wall Pilates—control, concentration, flow, and precision—remain consistent with traditional Pilates.

- **Control** is a foundational principle in Wall Pilates. This means that every movement should be performed with careful intent. When practitioners focus on controlling their movements, they can ensure they are executing each one correctly and safely. The wall acts as a supportive tool here. By using the wall, individuals can maintain proper alignment and posture more easily. For example, when doing leg lifts or stretching exercises, the wall can provide support, allowing practitioners to focus on executing the movement without worrying about losing their balance. As a result, this leads to better muscle engagement and reduces the risk of injury.

- Another essential principle in Wall Pilates is **concentration** . Practicing concentration involves fully engaging both the mind and body during each exercise. It helps individuals stay focused on their movements and the muscles they are working. To improve concentration, practitioners can start by setting aside distractions. This may mean finding a quiet space to practice or turning off devices that may interrupt their session. Once a focused environment is established, they can pay attention to their breath, the sensations in their body, and the specific movements they are performing. For instance, while performing a roll-up exercise, focusing on the articulation of the spine can help enhance the effectiveness of the movement and maintain the body's coordination.

- **Flow** is a principle that emphasizes the importance of smooth transitions between exercises. In Wall Pilates, creating flow is about connecting movements in a way that feels seamless and natural. This can improve overall workout efficiency and make the practice more enjoyable. To achieve this, practitioners can plan their routines in a way that the exercises naturally lead into one another. For example, a session could start with a wall push-up, transitioning smoothly into a wall squat, and then shifting to a wall stretch. By mapping out the routine ahead of time, practitioners can maintain a rhythm that keeps their body engaged and moving fluidly.

- **Precision** in Wall Pilates focuses on the accuracy of each movement. This principle encourages practitioners to target specific muscle groups effectively. Precision does not just mean making movements small or slight; it means ensuring that every motion serves a purpose. For example, while performing a wall plank, attention should be paid to how the core is engaged, how the arms are positioned, and how the legs maintain alignment. Individuals might find it helpful to perform each exercise in front of a mirror or record their movements, allowing them to identify areas where they can improve their precision. Practicing with this level of awareness can lead to better outcomes and results.

Connection to Mindfulness

These principles not only enhance physical fitness but also cultivate mindfulness. Wall Pilates encourages practitioners to be present and aware during their workouts. The focus required for each movement fosters a meditative state, promoting mental clarity and reducing stress. Mindfulness in Wall Pilates is further enhanced through controlled breathing patterns, which synchronize with movements, helping individuals stay centered and grounded.

Wall Pilates also incorporates mindfulness through the use of a dedicated space. Practitioners create an environment that is free from distractions, allowing them to connect deeper with their bodies and thoughts. This intentional setting enhances the overall experience, making it easier for individuals to focus on their movements. When the mind is clear and the space is serene, each session becomes an opportunity to explore both physical and mental boundaries. The walls themselves can serve as a tool for reflection, reminding practitioners to align not just their bodies but their minds as well.

Another aspect of mindfulness in Wall Pilates is the attention to alignment and form. Each movement requires a conscious effort to maintain proper posture and engage the right muscles. This level of focus pushes individuals to listen to their bodies, creating a dialogue between mind and movement. By paying close attention to how every position feels, practitioners learn to trust their instincts and become attuned to their own needs. This self-awareness builds a stronger connection to the concepts of mindfulness, allowing them to carry this awareness beyond their exercise routine.

Mindfulness is also nurtured by the rhythms of Wall Pilates. Many sessions are structured around a series of movements that flow into one another, creating a sense of continuity. This rhythm can allow practitioners to enter a flow state, where thoughts become less scattered, and the world outside fades away. As they move, they can lose themselves in the sequence, the pace of the workout guiding them to a state of calmness. The predictability of this rhythm provides a comforting backdrop, allowing individuals to immerse themselves in the experience fully.

The Principles of Wall Pilates

Wall Pilates goes beyond just a regular workout; it is a practice that encourages participants to connect with their bodies and minds on a deeper level. When we practice Wall Pilates, we are not merely going through the motions. Instead, we are learning to be present, focusing on our physical experience in the moment. This approach prompts us to set aside our daily distractions, such as worries about work or personal tasks, allowing us to immerse ourselves fully in the exercise.

Creating a mind-body connection is crucial in any physical activity, but Wall Pilates particularly emphasizes this concept. By being mindful during our workouts, we develop an awareness of our bodies that enriches the entire experience. This heightened awareness isn't just about feeling the physical sensations; it involves understanding how our bodies respond to various movements. As we engage in exercises, we start to notice subtle changes in our muscles and joints. An excellent example of this practice is during a wall roll-down. Here, we must focus on how each section of our spine stretches and how our muscles engage from our head to our toes.

Developing body awareness through Wall Pilates can significantly enhance our overall fitness journey. As we practice, we learn to listen to our bodies, recognizing where we may feel tension or discomfort. This is important because it allows us to adjust our movements accordingly. If we notice tightness in our shoulders during a particular exercise, we might modify our position to prevent injury. Being in tune with our bodies helps us appreciate what they can achieve and encourages us to treat them with care and respect.

In Wall Pilates, every movement has a purpose. This direct relationship encourages us to engage fully with each action we perform. For instance, consider a simple exercise like a wall squat. Instead of just sitting back into it, we should pay attention to how our legs align and how our core supports the squat. Are we breathing evenly? Are we maintaining proper posture? Asking these questions while performing the exercise helps keep our minds focused, ensuring we gain the maximum benefit from our practice.

One of the challenges in many exercise routines is allowing our minds to let go of external thoughts and pressures. Wall Pilates encourages us to release those thoughts as we move. By focusing on our present sensations and breathing, we create a space where stress and anxiety can diminish. This experience can be very liberating. Understanding that our practice is a judgment-free zone helps us enjoy the movement more. We realize that the goal isn't perfection but rather connection, progress, and personal growth.

Discovering Strength Through Control

Wall Pilates also emphasizes control in our movements. Unlike high-impact exercises, Wall Pilates allows us to move deliberately and at our own pace. This control helps us discover our inner strength. For example, when performing an exercise like the wall push-up, we can practice controlling our descent and ascent. We can choose to pause midway, focusing on the strength of our arms and core. This ability to control our movements not only builds strength but also reinforces our awareness of how our bodies function.

Cultivating Mindfulness Through Movement

The act of concentrating on each movement creates what can be described as a meditative state. During a Wall Pilates session, we can find clarity in our thoughts as we move. This clear state of mind can often lead to a reduction in stress levels. Many individuals find that after a workout, they feel lighter and more at ease. This transformation occurs because the body releases tension, and the mind becomes clearer of distractions. It is a simple yet effective way to unwind.

In Wall Pilates, the movements often require a level of precision. This precision is essential, as it helps individuals understand their limits and strengths better. For instance, maintaining proper alignment during a wall push-up can be challenging, but perfecting this can lead to improved strength over time. Each time we focus on alignment, we are practicing patience and acceptance, which are vital components of mindfulness.

Breathing Patterns and Centering

Another important aspect of mindfulness in Wall Pilates is the control of breathing patterns. Breathing is a fundamental part of any exercise routine, but in Wall Pilates, it takes on an even greater significance. Each breath can be synchronized with our movements, creating a rhythm that enhances our focus. For example, inhaling when performing an extension and exhaling during a contraction can make the exercises more effective. This pattern not only supports physical performance but also keeps our minds centered.

Controlled breathing allows individuals to stay grounded. When we breathe deeply and mindfully, we create a space where stress cannot easily enter. For instance, as we breathe into a stretch, we open ourselves up to relaxation. This self-awareness, coupled with self-regulation of breath, helps us maintain a calm and composed mind throughout our practice

Accessibility Features

Wall Pilates also stands out for its adaptability across varying fitness levels. Whether someone is new to exercise or has been active for years, Wall Pilates can be tailored to meet individual needs. Beginners benefit from the support the wall provides, allowing them to build confidence and stability without feeling overwhelmed. More advanced practitioners can increase the intensity by adjusting the angle of their bodies or incorporating additional movements.

The structured nature of Wall Pilates ensures that exercises can be modified easily. For example, a basic wall sit can be transformed into a more challenging workout by adding arm movements or incorporating small weights. This adaptability makes Wall Pilates a sustainable and progressive exercise routine for everyone, regardless of age or physical condition.

Key Benefits for Physical and Mental Well-Being

Wall Pilates offers a range of health benefits extending across physical, mental, and social domains, making it an excellent choice for individuals of all ages and fitness levels. By focusing on improving flexibility, strength, balance, and overall well-being, Wall Pilates can be a transformative addition to your wellness routine.

Physical Benefits

- **Improved Flexibility:** One of the primary physical advantages of Wall Pilates is improved flexibility. Regular practice involves various stretching exercises that enhance muscle elasticity and joint mobility, important for maintaining a healthy range of motion, especially as we age. Improved flexibility not only aids in reducing stiffness but also minimizes the risk of injuries (Cleveland Clinic, 2023). This benefit is particularly significant for seniors who seek to retain independence and engage in daily activities without discomfort.

- **Strength:** Strength is another key area where Wall Pilates excels. The exercises target core muscles, including the abdomen, back, hips, and buttocks, thereby building a strong foundation for the body. Strengthening these muscles supports better posture, reduces lower back pain, and enhances overall stability (Cleveland Clinic, 2023). For beginner fitness enthusiasts, developing core strength through Wall Pilates adds a solid base for other physical activities, ensuring they undertake more intense workouts safely.

- **Balance:** Balance and coordination are critical components of physical health, particularly for older adults at a higher risk of falls. Wall Pilates helps improve proprioception—the sense of body position in space—by engaging multiple muscle groups harmoniously. Enhanced balance reduces the likelihood of falls and related injuries, fostering greater confidence in movement (Cleveland Clinic, 2023). For younger practitioners, better coordination translates to more effective performance in sports and daily tasks.

Mental Benefits

Beyond physical benefits, Wall Pilates significantly contributes to mental well-being. One of the most valued aspects is stress relief. The focused movements and controlled breathing techniques inherent in Wall Pilates encourage mindfulness, helping practitioners become more present and centered during sessions. This mindful approach can alleviate anxiety and reduce cortisol levels, promoting a sense of calm and relaxation (Lim & Hyun, 2021).

Increased mental clarity is another psychological advantage. Engaging in regular Wall Pilates sessions encourages better oxygen flow to the brain through deep, intentional breathing. This increased oxygenation supports cognitive function, improves focus, and sharpens decision-making abilities. For both seniors and beginners, cultivating mental clarity can enhance everyday life, from managing tasks with ease to enjoying leisure activities more fully.

Connection with Community

Social benefits also emerge from participating in Wall Pilates classes. Joining group sessions creates opportunities for social interaction, essential for emotional health. Building connections with fellow practitioners fosters a sense of community and belonging, which can mitigate feelings of loneliness and isolation. Social bonds formed in these settings often extend outside the class, contributing to a richer social life and supportive network.

Forming a community within Wall Pilates classes can also encourage accountability. Friends push each other to show up, celebrate milestones, and inspire consistency in practice. It's easier to commit when others watch your progress and cheer for your goals.

This supportive network helps individuals stay on track, as they soak in motivation from one another. It becomes less about individual achievement and more about collective success, where each person's growth boosts the entire group's spirit.

Holistic Approach

Viewing exercise as a key part of staying healthy is very important. Adding Wall Pilates to your daily routine should be seen as more than just working out; it's also about improving your overall health. This approach recognizes that physical fitness, mental health, and social relationships are all connected. A good wellness routine can combine Wall Pilates with other activities like walking, swimming, or yoga, along with practices that support mental and emotional well-being, such as meditation or keeping a journal.

Adopting Wall Pilates regularly can encourage healthier habits. For example, the discipline from Pilates can help you eat better and lead a balanced life. These good habits work together, where improvements in one area of health boost others, leading to a well-rounded and lasting approach to wellness.

Equipment Needed and Setting Up a Practice Space

Creating a conducive environment for Wall Pilates practice and understanding the minimal equipment needed is essential for those beginning or continuing their fitness journey. Establishing a dedicated space and ensuring you have the necessary tools can greatly enhance your experience.

Essential Equipment

First, let's focus on the essential equipment required for Wall Pilates. While Wall Pilates is relatively minimalist in terms of gear, there are certain items that can significantly improve your practice. The primary equipment includes a sturdy wall, a quality exercise mat, resistance bands, and perhaps a Pilates ball.

A sturdy wall serves as the main support for many exercises, allowing you to leverage your body weight effectively. It is the foundation of Wall Pilates workouts, providing stability and enabling various movements that enhance strength and flexibility. A quality exercise mat is another item. It offers comfort and protects your joints during floor exercises. Look for mats that are non-slip, thick enough to cushion your body, and easy to clean.

Resistance bands are versatile tools in Wall Pilates that help add resistance to movements, enhancing muscle engagement and strength building. They come in different levels of resistance, making them suitable for both beginners and advanced practitioners. Lastly, a Pilates ball can be used to add an element of instability to your exercises, further challenging your core and balance.

Setting Up a Space

Creating a dedicated practice area is vital for maintaining consistency and focus. Whether you're setting up at home or in a community setting, certain factors should be considered to optimize your environment. Start by assessing the available space in your home. Choose a spot that is well-ventilated and spacious enough to accommodate your movements and equipment comfortably. This could be a spare room, a corner of your living room, or even a section of your bedroom.

Noise and disturbance are key considerations when choosing a location. Select an area that minimizes distractions, allowing you to fully concentrate on your practice. A quiet environment helps you stay present and engaged with each movement, which is critical for reaping the benefits of Wall Pilates. If possible, choose a space with ample natural light. Natural light can uplift your mood and create a serene atmosphere, enhancing your overall experience.

Once you've identified your practice area, consider how you can personalize it to reflect your preferences. Personalization is more than just aesthetics; it's about creating a space that feels inviting and motivating. You might choose to decorate with inspiring artwork, add plants for a touch of nature, or play calming music to set the tone. These elements can make your practice more enjoyable and increase your commitment to regular sessions.

Digital Resources

The role of technology has become increasingly important in modern fitness routines, including Wall Pilates. Online classes offer flexibility and accessibility, allowing you to participate in guided sessions from the comfort of your home. Platforms like Zoom or specialized fitness apps provide access to experienced instructors who can guide you through exercises, offer modifications, and help you maintain proper form.

Community support is another valuable aspect of online resources. Engaging with a virtual community of fellow practitioners can provide motivation and accountability. Many online platforms have forums or social media groups where you can share progress, ask questions, and receive encouragement. This sense of belonging can be particularly beneficial for seniors or beginners, helping them stay committed and feel supported.

Personalization

Remember, the key to a sustainable Wall Pilates practice lies in nurturing a dynamic environment. Continuously evolve your space with new ideas and equipment as you grow. Aim to establish a space that feels personal to you—one that uplifts your spirits and keeps you engaged in your fitness journey. The more you experiment with you your studio setup, the more enjoyable and fulfilling your practice will become.

Consider reaching out to Pilates communities or forums, where you can share ideas and get feedback on how to optimize your space. Collaborating with others can provide fresh perspectives and inspiration. Creating a practice that is entirely yours will lead to a deeper connection with Wall Pilates. Embrace this evolution in your practice for a happier, healthier you.

Encouraging creativity in setting up your space can also play a significant role in making your Wall Pilates practice sustainable. Think about how your space can evolve with your practice. For example, you might start with basic equipment and gradually introduce new elements as you become more comfortable with the exercises. Keep an open mind and allow your environment to grow and adapt alongside your fitness journey.

Different Fitness Levels and Modifications

Wall Pilates is a flexible way to get fit, making it good for people of all ages and fitness levels. It's important to know the different fitness skills of those who want to join, so everyone can practice Wall Pilates safely and effectively.

Understanding Fitness Levels

Individuals new to physical activity or those with limited strength and flexibility may require modifications to basic exercises to prevent injury and build confidence. For example, a beginner might start with simpler movements such as wall-assisted squats or gentle stretches using the wall for support. These modifications maintain the integrity of the exercise while reducing strain on muscles and joints.

On the other hand, more experienced practitioners might seek to challenge themselves further by incorporating advanced variations of exercises into their routines. For instance, they could progress to moves like wall planks or single-leg balances, which demand greater stability and strength.

Modifications for Safety

To safely modify exercises for different capabilities, it is essential to listen to your body and avoid pushing beyond comfort levels. Begin with foundational exercises to establish a solid base and gradually introduce more complex movements as confidence and strength grow. Use the wall as a supportive tool to maintain proper alignment and balance throughout the practice.

When you do modify exercises, never hesitate to ask for help. Whether you are in a gym or a yoga studio, instructors can provide invaluable insights into correct form and adaptations suitable for your capabilities. They can suggest alternative movements or even offer tips for ensuring that you're practicing safely. This support can give you greater confidence as you explore new exercises.

Finally, remember that modifying exercises allows you to create a workout routine tailored specifically for you. It's a journey to finding out what your body can do, and being in tune with yourself is a vital part of that journey. Treat each workout as an opportunity to learn more about what feels good and what promotes your physical well-being. In turn, this mindset can turn exercise into a more enjoyable and sustainable habit in your daily life.

Progress Tracking

Progress tracking plays a vital role in ensuring continuous improvement and motivation. One practical tip for gauging progress is to maintain a journal of your workouts, noting the exercises performed, duration, and perceived difficulty. This record helps identify patterns and areas where you have improved or need further attention. Additionally, periodically measuring your flexibility, strength, and balance can provide tangible evidence of your progress.

Adjusting routines based on these observations allows for a tailored approach that meets evolving fitness goals. For instance, if you notice significant improvements in your core strength, you might decide to incorporate more challenging core exercises or increase the duration of your routine. Similarly, if flexibility advancements are slow, incorporating additional stretching sessions may be beneficial.

Community Support

Community support significantly enhances the Wall Pilates experience. Engaging with others who share similar fitness goals provides encouragement, accountability, and a sense of belonging. Local fitness centers, community classes, or online forums dedicated to Wall Pilates offer opportunities to connect with fellow practitioners. Sharing experiences and challenges with others fosters a supportive environment that motivates continued participation and growth.

Participating in group classes led by certified instructors can also ensure correct form and technique, reducing the risk of injury. Instructors can provide personalized feedback and suggest modifications based on individual needs, further customizing the practice. Attending workshops or training sessions can deepen your understanding of Wall Pilates, allowing you to explore more advanced techniques under professional guidance.

Leveraging technology can enhance community engagement. Apps and online platforms offer virtual classes, instructional videos, and social networking features that connect practitioners worldwide. Engaging in these virtual communities enables sharing of tips, success stories, and motivational content, creating a dynamic and interactive learning environment.

Moving Forward with Wall Pilates

This chapter has introduced the core principles and advantages of Wall Pilates, highlighting its historical background and evolution from traditional Pilates. By incorporating the wall as a supportive tool, Wall Pilates offers stability and resistance, making it accessible to individuals of all ages and fitness levels. The emphasis on control, concentration, flow, and precision ensures that practitioners can perform movements with mindful intent, promoting both physical health and mental well-being.

As we transition from the foundational concepts introduced in this chapter, let us delve into foundational exercises, where readers will discover essential wall-supported stretches that enhance flexibility and promote relaxation, serving as a vital step in their Wall Pilates journey.

Chapter 2
Getting Started:
Foundational Exercises

N ext, we'll set the stage for a balanced and effective practice. Proper alignment and posture are critical elements that ensure the body's movements are efficient, minimize the risk of injury, and maximize the benefits derived from each exercise. This chapter delves into the principles of maintaining a neutral spine, appropriate foot placement, and executing alignment checks to safeguard against common mistakes. It provides detailed insights on how to use visual and tactile feedback for self-assessment, ensuring that beginners build a solid foundation from the outset. Emphasis is also placed on core activation techniques that not only enhance stability but also support overall movement efficiency.

Proper Alignment and Posture

Establishing proper alignment and posture is crucial for an effective Wall Pilates session. Good alignment enhances movement efficiency, lowers the chance of injury, and amplifies the benefits of each exercise.

Neutral Spine

Understanding neutral spine is crucial for maintaining proper alignment in Wall Pilates. The neutral spine position involves maintaining the natural curves of the spine: a slight curve in the lumbar region (lower back), a slight curve in the thoracic region (mid-back), and another slight curve in the cervical region (neck). This position helps distribute forces evenly across the vertebrae and surrounding muscles, which enhances the effectiveness of exercises and prevents strain.

When practicing Wall Pilates, always be aware of your spine's alignment. Imagine drawing a straight line from the top of your head down through your tailbone; this visualization can help maintain a neutral spine throughout movements.

To confirm your neutral spine, start with grounding your feet firmly on the floor, ensuring they are hip-width apart. Engage your core muscles slightly to support your lower back. As you breathe in, focus on bringing your shoulders away from your ears, allowing them to relax.

Next, try to keep your chin parallel to the floor. Imagine holding a tennis ball between your chin and chest. If the ball falls, it means your head is too far forward or back. Keep your neck long and in line with your spine.

Foot Placement

Foot placement is crucial for maintaining stability during Wall Pilates exercises. When practicing these movements, your feet serve as the foundation for your body. If your footing is not correct, it can lead to misalignment and affect your overall performance. So, let's dive into why proper foot positioning matters and how it impacts your workout.

Proper Positioning for Stability

To achieve a stable and effective workout, your feet should generally be hip-width apart and parallel to each other. This positioning creates a solid base of support, allowing your body to function effectively. For instance, when you stand with your feet hip-width apart, your legs align with your hips. This alignment is essential because it helps distribute weight evenly and reduces strain on your joints. If your feet are too close together or too far apart, it can destabilize your posture, making some exercises more challenging and potentially harmful.

When you stand in this proper foot position, you create a more balanced stance. A balanced stance is important in Wall Pilates, where you often engage in movements that require control and precision. Imagine doing a leg lift or a wall squat. If your feet are placed correctly, you are less likely to wobble or lose your balance, which allows you to focus on the exercise itself rather than worrying about falling over.

Engaging the Right Muscles

In Wall Pilates, the wall acts as a helpful guide for foot placement. It provides a visual and physical reference point, making it easier to find your footing. When you press the soles of your feet firmly into the floor or against the wall, you engage multiple muscle groups, including those in your legs and core. This engagement is key to enhancing your stability and control during exercises.

For example, when performing a Wall Pilates exercise like the wall push-up, pressing your feet into the ground helps activate your quads and glutes. These muscles play a significant role in supporting your body. As they engage, you may notice that you feel more grounded and stable. This firm connection to the ground helps you maintain alignment, making it less likely that you will shift or lose your form while executing the move.

Importance of Balance and Control

Control is a major component of Wall Pilates exercises. Proper foot placement allows you to maintain control throughout your movements. When you shift your weight correctly and align your body with your feet, each exercise becomes smoother and more fluid. Take the Wall Pilates leg press as an example. When your feet are in the right position, pushing against the wall feels more comfortable and efficient.

To practice control, focus on how your feet are positioned before you begin an exercise. Make sure they are parallel and hip-width apart. This will not only help with balance but also allow you to transfer weight evenly across your feet. Poor foot placement can lead to unintended movements that may strain your muscles or joints. Therefore, keep reiterating the importance of checking your foot placement as part of your warm-up routine.

Alignment Checks

For beginners, conducting alignment checks is essential to ensure they are performing exercises correctly. One useful technique is to use a mirror to observe and adjust your posture. Pay attention to key indicators such as the position of the shoulders, hips, knees, and feet. Another method is to perform tactile checks, such as placing a hand on the lower back to feel if there is too much arching or flattening.

Another way to conduct alignment checks is to engage in partner assessments. Having a trusted friend or instructor observe your movements can provide valuable feedback. They can highlight any misalignments you may not notice, such as asymmetrical movements or unequal weight distribution. It's essential to communicate openly with your partner about what to look for. Encourage them to gently point out areas for improvement. This collaborative approach fosters a supportive environment where both individuals can learn from each other, further enhancing their skills.

One more helpful technique is to utilize props during practice. Items like foam rollers, yoga blocks, or resistance bands can offer support and guidance in achieving proper alignment. For instance, placing a yoga block under the hands during a downward dog can help maintain correct shoulder positioning. Similarly, using a foam roller for muscle release can alleviate tension, allowing for a more natural alignment. Experimenting with these tools can deepen your understanding of alignment while adding variety to your routine.

Engaging in these self-assessments regularly can help identify and correct misalignments before they become ingrained habits. Incorporating breath awareness can also aid in maintaining proper alignment. Breathing deeply and evenly encourages relaxation and alignment of the spine, thereby supporting overall posture.

Common Alignment Mistakes to Avoid

It's also important to recognize common alignment mistakes that could hinder progress in Wall Pilates practice. One frequent error is allowing the shoulders to round forward, which can lead to tension in the neck and upper back. To avoid this, think about gently pulling the shoulder blades down and together, opening up the chest while keeping the shoulders relaxed. Similarly, hyperextending the lower back is a common mistake, particularly when trying to maintain an upright posture. This can be corrected by engaging the abdominal muscles and lifting the tailbone slightly toward the pelvis to maintain a neutral spine.

Another typical misalignment issue is improper head positioning, often seen as tilting the head too far forward or backward. The head should be aligned with the spine, maintaining a straight line from the crown to the tailbone. Imagine lengthening the neck upward, as if being gently pulled by a string attached to the top of the head; this can help keep the head in proper alignment. Don't forget to be mindful of the hips' position. Tilting the pelvis too far forward or backward can disrupt the neutral spine alignment. Ensuring the hips are squared and level is key to maintaining balance and stability.

Awareness of posture extends beyond just the spine and hips; it includes the knees and ankles as well. The knees should remain soft, not locked, to allow for natural shock absorption by the leg muscles. Keeping the knees aligned with the toes ensures that the entire leg functions harmoniously during movements, preventing unnecessary strain on the knee joints. Moreover, distributing weight evenly across the feet is critical. Avoid placing excessive pressure on the heels or balls of the feet; instead, aim to have even contact with the ground through all parts of the foot.

Core Activation Techniques

Understanding the core involves recognizing that it is not just about having visible abs, but rather a complex group of muscles that reside in the midsection. These muscles include the rectus abdominis, transverse abdominis, internal and external obliques, and the muscles of the pelvic floor and lower back. Essentially, the core acts as a central support structure for the entire body, facilitating movement and maintaining balance.

The core muscles play a crucial role in almost every bodily movement. They provide a stable base for motion, ensuring that activities such as walking, lifting, or even sitting are performed with minimal strain on other parts of the body. Properly engaging these muscles helps maintain spinal alignment and reduces the risk of injury. By understanding the components and functions of the core, practitioners can appreciate the necessity of strengthening these muscles through targeted exercises.

Breathing is an essential component of effective core engagement. The diaphragm, a dome-shaped muscle located beneath the lungs, plays a significant role in breathing and core stability. When you inhale deeply, the diaphragm contracts and flattens, creating space for the lungs to expand. This action generates intra-abdominal pressure, which supports the spine and stabilizes the trunk during movements.

To activate the core effectively, it is important to synchronize breathing with specific muscle contractions. For instance, when performing an exercise like a plank, one should take a deep breath in through the nose, allowing the abdomen to expand slightly. As you exhale through the mouth, gently draw your navel toward your spine, engaging the deep core muscles. This technique not only strengthens the core but also ensures that the exercises are performed safely and efficiently.

Exercises designed specifically for core activation are simple yet highly effective. Here are a few foundational movements:

1. **Abdominal Bracing** : Lie on your back with your knees bent. Tighten your abdominal muscles by pulling your navel toward your spine while

maintaining a neutral spine position. Hold this contraction for 10 seconds and repeat 10 times.

1. **Alternating Leg Marching** : Begin in the same position as abdominal bracing. Perform abdominal bracing while lifting each leg about 12 inches off the ground in a slow, controlled manner. Alternate legs, performing 10 reps on each side per set.

1. **Dead Bug** : Lie on your back with your knees and hips bent at 90 degrees. Perform abdominal bracing while partially extending one leg at a time. Alternate legs, aiming for 10 reps on each side.

1. **Partial Sit-Ups** : With your knees bent and hands on your thighs, tighten your abs and lift your upper back off the floor while sliding your hands up your thighs. Hold the lifted position for two seconds, then return to the starting position. Perform 10 reps per set.

These exercises are particularly beneficial for beginners because they target the deep core muscles without placing excessive stress on the spine.

Progressions for core strength involve gradually increasing the difficulty of the exercises as core stability improves. For example, once basic abdominal bracing becomes easier, one can progress to more advanced movements such as the bridge exercise. Here are some suggested progressions:

1. **Partial Bridge to Full Bridge** : Start with a partial bridge by lying on your back with knees bent and feet flat on the floor. Tighten your abs and lift your hips and buttocks off the floor, holding the position for five seconds before lowering back down. Gradually increase the hold time to 10 seconds as tolerated. Once comfortable with the partial bridge, progress to a full bridge by lifting the hips higher.

1. **Bridge with Exercise Ball** : Lie on your back with your calves resting on an exercise ball. Tighten your abs and lift your hips and buttocks in a controlled manner, avoiding hyperextension of the spine. Hold for two seconds before returning to the starting position. Perform 10 reps per set.

1. **Alternating Arm & Leg Lifts** : Lie on your stomach with a pillow underneath your hips. Tighten your abs and alternate lifting opposite arms and legs, holding each lift for one second. This exercise strengthens the lower back and improves overall core stability.

1. **Hands & Knees Alternating Leg Lifts** : Assume a hands-and-knees position with hands under shoulders and knees under hips. Tighten your abs and slowly lift one leg at a time, holding

each lift for one second. Alternate sides, performing 10 reps on each leg per set.

1. **Hands & Knees Alternating Opposite Arm & Leg Lifts** : From the same starting position, extend the opposite arm and leg while tightening the core. Hold for one second and then alternate sides. This exercise enhances coordination and balance while targeting multiple core muscles.

Incorporating these progressions into your routine allows for continuous improvement in core strength and stability. It is essential to perform each exercise with proper form, emphasizing controlled movements and consistent core engagement.

By focusing on understanding the core, practicing effective breathing techniques, and incorporating specific exercises, beginners and seniors alike can build a strong foundation of core strength. Progressions ensure that as strength improves, challenges increase, leading to greater stability and support in daily activities and advanced exercises alike.

Introduction to Basic Wall-Supported Stretches

The benefits of wall-supported stretching are numerous. Firstly, utilizing a wall for support significantly enhances stretch effectiveness. The stability provided by the wall allows practitioners to maintain proper alignment throughout the exercise. This stability helps prevent common mistakes such as improper posture or misalignment, which can reduce the effectiveness of the stretch and potentially lead to injury. The wall acts as a resistance tool, enabling a deeper stretch that might be harder to achieve otherwise. For seniors looking to maintain their range of motion or beginner fitness enthusiasts aiming to build flexibility, wall-supported stretches offer a controlled environment where they can comfortably push their limits.

Introducing wall-supported stretches into your fitness routine can improve flexibility and encourage relaxation. These stretches enhance movement and help calm the mind, making them a great addition to any wellness plan. Let's explore some key wall-supported stretches designed to be beginner-friendly yet effective:

1. **Quadriceps Stretch** : Stand near a wall for balance. Grasp your ankle and gently pull your heel towards your buttocks until you feel a stretch along the front of your thigh. Keep your knees close together, and ensure your abdominal muscles stay engaged to avoid sagging. Hold the position for about 30 seconds before switching legs. This stretch alleviates tightness in the

quadriceps and can help improve your overall leg mobility (A Guide to Basic Stretches, 2023).

1. **Hip Flexor Stretch** : Start by kneeling on one knee with the other foot planted in front of you, creating a 90-degree angle at both knees. Use the wall or a piece of sturdy furniture for support. Lean forward slightly, transferring weight onto the front leg until you feel a stretch in the hip flexor of the back leg. Hold this position for 30 seconds before switching sides. This stretch is vital for those who spend a lot of time sitting, as it helps open up the hips and enhance mobility.

1. **Iliotibial Band Stretch (ITB)** : Stand beside a wall and cross one leg over the other at the ankles. Extend the arm closest to the wall overhead and lean towards the wall. You should feel a stretch along the outer part of your hip and thigh. Hold for about 30 seconds and switch sides. The ITB stretch is beneficial for runners and walkers, as it targets a band of tissue that is often prone to tightness.

1. **Calf Stretch** : Position yourself at arm's length from a wall. Place one foot behind the other, keeping the back knee straight and the heel on the ground. Slowly bend the front knee while pressing the back heel into the floor. Hold for 30 seconds before switching legs. This stretch helps in relieving tension in the calf muscles and

improving ankle flexibility (A Guide to Basic Stretches, 2023).

Incorporating breath with stretches plays a critical role in enhancing the benefits of these exercises. Breathing deeply during stretches increases oxygen flow to the muscles, facilitates relaxation, and can make the stretch more effective. As you stretch, inhale deeply through your nose, filling your lungs completely. Exhale slowly and thoroughly, allowing your muscles to relax into the stretch. This mindful breathing practice not only helps deepen the stretch but also promotes a sense of calm and tranquility, making your stretching session a holistic experience.

Safety Tips

Safe stretching practices are very important for preventing injuries and getting the most out of your routines. When you stretch properly, you can improve your flexibility, reduce muscle tension, and enhance your overall performance. However, improper stretching can lead to strains or other injuries. To make sure you are stretching safely, there are some essential guidelines to follow.

1. **Warm Up** : Always warm up before stretching with light activities like walking or gentle jogging to increase blood flow to the muscles. This

prepares the body for more extensive stretching, reducing the risk of strains.

1. **Stretch Gently** : Avoid bouncing or jerking movements while stretching. Instead, move slowly and smoothly into each stretch until you feel a gentle pull. Bouncing can cause micro-tears in the muscles, leading to soreness and potential injury.

1. **Tune into Your Body:** Notice the sensations in your body while performing each stretch. If you experience sharp pain, ease off immediately. Stretching should never be painful; instead, it should create a comfortable tension.

1. **Hold and Breathe** : Maintain each stretch for about 30 seconds, ensuring you breathe steadily throughout. Holding your breath can create unnecessary tension and reduce the effectiveness of the stretch.

1. **Consistency** : Incorporate stretching into your routine regularly, ideally after workouts when the muscles are warm. Aim to stretch major muscle groups at least 2-3 times per week for optimal results.

1. **Comfortable Positioning** : Make sure your positioning is comfortable and supported to avoid straining other parts of your body. For instance, if a stretch requires kneeling, use a towel or cushion

under your knee for added comfort (A Guide to Basic Stretches, 2023).

Bringing It All Together

This chapter has provided a comprehensive overview of essential Wall Pilates exercises, emphasizing the importance of proper alignment, core activation, and wall-supported stretches. By understanding and maintaining a neutral spine, practitioners can enhance their efficiency and reduce injury risks. The chapter has detailed various techniques to ensure correct posture and alignment, such as using mirrors for self-assessment and observing common mistakes to avoid.

The focus on core activation underscores the necessity of engaging the muscles in the midsection for stability and support during exercises. With practical guidance on breathing techniques and fundamental movements, both seniors and beginner fitness enthusiasts alike can build a strong foundation for their Wall Pilates practice. Incorporating wall-supported stretches further complements this routine by enhancing flexibility and promoting relaxation. By following these guidelines, practitioners can confidently progress in their fitness journey, ensuring safe and effective workouts.

Building on these foundational stretches, the next chapter invites you to explore a diverse array of Wall Pilates exercises that specifically target key muscle groups, enhancing your strength and conditioning in both the upper and lower body.

Chapter 3
Strength Training with Wall Pilates

Building muscular strength through Wall Pilates offers a practical and effective method to improve overall body health. Utilizing the wall for support in exercises enhances stability, making it easier for seniors to preserve functional fitness and for newcomers to establish their workout routines. By focusing on specific muscle groups with gentle movements, participants can build strength while minimizing stress on their joints, making this approach suitable for individuals with varying fitness levels.

Upper body strength exercises

Upper body strength plays a pivotal role in our daily activities and overall fitness. Whether it's lifting groceries, reaching for an item on a high shelf, or maintaining good posture while sitting at a desk, strong upper body muscles are essential. For seniors looking to maintain functional strength and flexibility, or beginners seeking to establish a consistent fitness routine, integrating targeted exercises such as Wall Pilates can be both beneficial and accessible.

Integrating these Wall Pilates exercises into your regular fitness routine can help you build and maintain upper body strength, which is essential for overall wellness. It's important to remember that progress may vary between individuals, and it's always advisable to consult a fitness professional to evaluate your fitness level and ensure that these exercises are tailored to your specific needs.

In addition to enhancing muscular strength, these exercises also offer the benefit of improved flexibility and balance. Regular practice can lead to better posture, reduced risk of injuries, and increased confidence in performing daily tasks. The low-impact nature of Wall Pilates makes it suitable for individuals of all ages and fitness levels, providing a safe and effective way to stay active.

Wall Push-Ups

One effective exercise to improve upper body strength is the Wall Push-Up. This variation of the traditional push-up uses the wall as support, making it easier for individuals who may find floor push-ups too challenging. To perform a Wall Push-Up, stand facing the wall with your feet hip-width apart and about a foot away from the wall. Place your palms flat against the wall at shoulder height, slightly wider than shoulder-width apart. Slowly bend your elbows out, not down, to lower your body towards the wall, keeping your back straight and your core engaged. Push back to the starting position by straightening your arms. This exercise primarily targets the chest, shoulders, and triceps, helping to build strength in these areas without putting excessive strain on the joints.

Advanced Variation

- A variation of the Wall Push-Up is the Incline Wall Push-Up. This exercise is similar but adds a different angle to the movement. To perform the Incline Wall Push-Up, you follow the same initial steps as the standard version. However, you elevate your feet on a step or a low bench. This position shifts your body angle, making the exercise slightly more challenging as it requires additional strength from the chest, shoulders, and core to stabilize. The higher your feet are, the harder the exercise becomes. It's an excellent progression for those who have mastered the regular Wall Push-Up and are looking to enhance their upper body strength further.

Wall Arm Raises

This movement focuses on strengthening the shoulders and upper back, which are crucial for maintaining good posture and reducing the risk of shoulder injuries. To perform Wall Arm Raises, stand with your back against the wall and your feet flat on the ground. Keep your arms by your sides with your palms facing forward. Slowly raise your arms to shoulder height, keeping them straight and in contact with the wall. Hold the position for a few seconds, then lower your arms back down. Repeat this motion, ensuring that your back remains flat against the wall throughout the exercise. By consistently practicing Wall Arm Raises, you can improve shoulder mobility and upper back strength, contributing to better posture and reduced muscle tension.

Seated Wall Press

For those who may have difficulty standing for long periods, the Seated Wall Press offers an excellent alternative. This exercise allows you to engage your upper body muscles while seated, providing stability and support. To perform the Seated Wall Press, sit on a chair or stool with your back against the wall and your feet flat on the ground. Place your hands on the wall at shoulder height, with your elbows bent at a 90-degree angle. Push against the wall, extending your arms forward. Hold the press for a few seconds before returning to the starting position. This exercise targets the chest, shoulders, and triceps, and can be easily adjusted to different fitness levels by varying the intensity of the press.

Wall Tricep Dips

The Wall Tricep Dip is another gentle yet effective exercise that specifically targets the triceps, the muscles located at the back of the upper arm. Strong triceps are important for activities like pushing open a door or getting up from a seated position. To perform Wall Tricep Dips, stand with your back against the wall and your feet a few inches away from it. Place your hands on the wall at hip height, with your fingers pointing downward. Bend your elbows to lower your body slightly, engaging the triceps. Push back up to the starting position by straightening your arms. This controlled movement helps to strengthen and tone the triceps while minimizing stress on the wrists and shoulders.

Advanced Variation

- An advanced variation of the Wall Tricep Dip can be performed by elevating your feet on a sturdy surface, like a low bench or a step. This adjustment increases the difficulty, as it requires greater strength and stability. With your feet raised, position your hands on the wall in the same way as before but lean slightly forward. This angle shifts more weight onto your triceps and engages your core muscles more effectively. As you lower your body, focus on maintaining a straight line from your head to your feet. It's important to control the movement, ensuring you don't drop too low, which could strain your shoulders.

- To enhance the workout, you can add pauses at the bottom of the movement. Engage your triceps fully by holding the dip position for a second or two before pressing back up. This added time under tension helps to build strength and endurance in the muscles. Remember to breathe steadily throughout the exercise. Inhale as you lower yourself and exhale as you push back to the starting position. Incorporating these pauses not only challenges your triceps but also helps you develop focus and control.

- Another way to advance this exercise is to perform the Wall Tricep Dip with one leg suspended in the air. While in the starting position, extend one leg straight out in front of you while resting the other foot on the ground. This adjustment requires more core engagement, stabilizing your body while you dip. Make sure to switch legs after a set to ensure both sides develop equally. As you get comfortable, consider increasing the duration of the leg lift, which will further test your balance and strength.

Lower body strength exercises

Lower body strength plays a vital role in our overall health and mobility. As we age, it becomes increasingly important to maintain strong muscles in our legs and glutes. This strength helps us keep our balance and prevents falls, which can be particularly dangerous for older adults. Strong muscles in these areas support our posture and allow for easier movement during daily activities, such as walking, climbing stairs, or even getting up from a chair.

When we think about the muscles in our lower body, we usually consider the quadriceps, hamstrings, calves, and glutes. Each of these muscle groups contributes to our stability and mobility. For example, the quadriceps help us extend our knees and provide support when standing up. The hamstrings play a crucial role in bending our knees and controlling our movements. The calves help with walking and balance, while the glutes are essential for standing, walking, and climbing stairs. Together, these muscles create a strong foundation that is necessary for a healthy and active lifestyle.

For those new to fitness, as well as aging adults, exercises that incorporate wall support can be highly effective as they offer stability and reduce the risk of injury. Below are several Wall Pilates exercises designed to enhance lower body strength for all fitness levels.

Wall Squats

Wall squats are a foundational exercise to strengthen the legs and glutes. To perform wall squats, stand with your back against a wall and feet shoulder-width apart. Slowly slide down the wall by bending your knees while keeping your back pressed firmly against the surface. Lower yourself until your thighs are parallel to the ground, ensuring your knees do not extend beyond your toes. Hold this position for a few seconds before returning to the starting position. Repeat this movement for several sets, gradually increasing the duration and intensity as you become more comfortable.

The wall squat is particularly beneficial because it engages multiple muscle groups, including the quadriceps, hamstrings, and glutes. This exercise helps build endurance and strength, which translates into improved performance in daily tasks like climbing stairs or lifting groceries. The wall provides support, making it an excellent choice for beginners or those with balance issues.

Calf Raises Against the Wall

Calf raises are another essential exercise that targets the muscles in the lower legs. Stand tall with your back against the wall and feet hip-width apart. Press your hands gently against the wall for support.

Slowly rise onto the balls of your feet, lifting your heels off the ground as high as possible. Hold this position briefly before lowering your heels back down. Repeat for several repetitions, focusing on a slow and controlled motion.

This exercise strengthens the calf muscles, improving overall stability and helping to prevent ankle injuries. Strong calves also contribute to better balance, particularly during activities like walking and running. As with wall squats, using the wall for support makes calf raises accessible to individuals of all fitness levels.

Side Leg Raises with Wall Support

Side leg raises are effective for strengthening the hip abductors, muscles located on the outer side of the hips. These muscles are key players in maintaining lateral stability and balance. To perform side leg raises, stand next to a wall and place one hand on the wall for support. Lift the outer leg sideways as high as comfortable while keeping the leg straight. Lower it back down slowly and repeat. Switch sides after completing a set.

Strengthening the hip abductors helps improve balance and coordination, reducing the risk of falls. This exercise is especially useful for seniors who may experience a natural decline in muscle strength and flexibility with age. The wall provides necessary support, allowing for correct form and reducing the likelihood of strain or injury.

Wall Sit

The wall sit is an isometric exercise that builds lower body endurance. To perform a wall sit, stand with your back against the wall and feet about two feet away from the wall. Slide down into a seated position, ensuring your thighs are parallel to the floor and your knees are directly above your ankles. Hold this position for as long as possible, then slowly rise back up to the starting position.

Wall sits effectively engage the quadriceps, hamstrings, glutes, and even the core muscles. This exercise enhances muscular endurance, which is beneficial for prolonged periods of standing or walking. By supporting the back, the wall decreases the risk of improper form, making it ideal for all fitness levels.

Full-body integration movements

Combining upper and lower body exercises in Wall Pilates offers a holistic approach to strength training, engaging multiple muscle groups simultaneously. This method promotes balanced muscular development, enhances functional fitness, and reduces the risk of injury. The integration of complementary movements for both the upper and lower body ensures a comprehensive workout that supports overall wellness.

Incorporating these combined movements into a regular fitness routine can significantly enhance overall strength and functionality. Each exercise is designed to work multiple muscle groups, ensuring a well-rounded workout. Wall Pilates is particularly beneficial for seniors who aim to maintain functional strength, as well as beginners who seek a structured yet varied exercise regimen.

One of the primary benefits of combining upper and lower body exercises is the efficient use of workout time. By engaging multiple muscle groups simultaneously, individuals can achieve a full-body workout in less time compared to isolating each muscle group. This efficiency is especially valuable for those with busy schedules or limited time for exercise. Working various muscle groups together helps raise the heart rate, providing cardiovascular benefits alongside strength training.

Moreover, these compound movements mimic everyday activities, leading to improved functional fitness. For instance, the coordination required for Lateral Wall Lunges with Reach reflects actions such as picking up objects from the floor or reaching for items on high shelves. Engaging in such multi-joint exercises prepares the body for real-life physical demands, reducing the likelihood of injuries and enhancing overall quality of life.

Combining upper and lower body exercises also fosters better muscle coordination and synergy. When multiple muscles work together, it trains the nervous system to coordinate and control movements effectively. This improved neuromuscular coordination translates to smoother and more efficient movements in daily life, contributing to overall functional agility.

Wall Pilates Roll Down

The Wall Pilates Roll Down is an essential exercise that engages the entire body while emphasizing spinal articulation. Start by standing with your back against the wall. Slowly roll down, vertebra by vertebra, until your hands reach as close to the floor as possible. This movement stretches the spine, activates the core muscles, and increases flexibility in the hamstrings. It's a gentle yet effective way to prepare the body for more dynamic movements, making it a perfect warm-up exercise.

Wall Leg Lifts with Arm Extensions

Next, the Wall Leg Lifts with Arm Extensions combine leg and arm motions to engage the core extensively. Position yourself with one side of your body against the wall, stabilizing with the opposite hand. Lift your outer leg to hip height while extending the arm on the same side overhead. This exercise not only targets the legs and shoulders but also requires the core to stabilize the body, enhancing balance and coordination.

Lateral Wall Lunges with Reach

Lateral Wall Lunges with Reach provide a functional movement pattern that integrates lower and upper body engagement. Stand with one side facing the wall, feet shoulder-width apart. Step out into a lunge position, ensuring your knee aligns with your ankle. As you lower into the lunge, extend the arm nearest to the wall overhead and slightly across your body. This move challenges the thighs, glutes, and obliques, while the reaching motion incorporates the shoulder and stretches the torso. It's an excellent exercise for improving mobility and functional strength, which are vital for daily activities such as reaching and bending.

Wall Supported Plan with Arm Row

The Wall Supported Plank with Arm Row is another powerful exercise that combines stability with dynamic upper body movements. Begin in a plank position with your feet against the wall, maintaining a straight line from head to heels. Lift one arm off the ground and perform a rowing motion, bringing the elbow past your torso. This exercise engages the core, glutes, and shoulders while also promoting strength in the upper back. The stability required for the plank position also strengthens the lower body and improves overall balance.

Techniques for Increasing Intensity

Wall Pilates exercises are adaptable and can be modified to suit different fitness levels. For seniors or individuals with mobility issues, these exercises offer the support necessary to perform movements safely. Beginners can also benefit from the wall's stability as they build confidence and strength. For example, the Wall Supported Plank can be modified by performing the plank on the knees, gradually progressing to a full plank as strength improves.

Incorporating variations into the routine can keep Wall Pilates engaging and challenging. For instance, adding twist movements at the wall can target the obliques, promoting a stronger core. Another variation includes wall push-ups, which can be modified to suit different fitness levels; beginners might start with wall push-ups at a slight angle while more advanced practitioners can transition to more challenging positions. Participants can also try unique exercises like wall sit with calf raises for a comprehensive lower body workout. These changes not only make the practice dynamic but also help in maintaining motivation and enjoyment.

Anyone can find their right pace and challenge themselves effectively. Each person's journey will look slightly different, but the principles of gradual progression and listening to one's body are universal. With each session, individuals will notice improvements, from enhanced strength to better balance and flexibility. Consistent practice, tailored to one's abilities, can lead to significant advancements in fitness levels and overall well-being.

Add Resistance Bands

Adding resistance bands to Wall Pilates can enhance the effectiveness of exercises. These bands provide extra resistance during movements, which helps build strength more efficiently. For example, when performing wall squats, attaching a resistance band around the thighs can increase the challenge. This added resistance engages more muscle groups, leading to better results over time. Individuals can start with lighter bands and gradually work their way up to heavier ones, ensuring that they can maintain proper form throughout their workout.

Increase the Range of Motion

Increasing the range of motion during exercises is another effective way to intensify a Wall Pilates practice. When performing movements like wall stretches or leg lifts, participants should focus on extending their limbs to their fullest capacity. This approach not only helps improve flexibility but also engages deeper muscle fibers. As confidence grows, individuals can incorporate movements that require more balance and control, like knee tucks or side leg lifts against the wall. These variations can assist in developing stronger core and leg muscles while supporting better functional fitness.

Extend Exercise Duration

Extending exercise duration is also a smart strategy for those looking to improve their Wall Pilates practice. Instead of sticking to a fixed amount of time, individuals can gradually increase their workout duration. For example, starting with 15-minute sessions and slowly working up to 30 or 45 minutes allows for progressive overload. This gradual approach helps to avoid injury and ensures that the body adapts appropriately. It's essential to listen to one's body and take breaks when needed. Incorporating longer sessions also allows for more variation, including warm-up, cool-down, and additional stretches.

Key Takeaways for Your Journey

This chapter has explored the significance of building muscular strength through targeted Wall Pilates exercises. By emphasizing both upper and lower body strength, these exercises provide a balanced approach to overall wellness. Upper body movements such as Wall Push-Ups, Wall Arm Raises, Seated Wall Presses, and Wall Tricep Dips help improve functional strength while ensuring joint safety. Similarly, lower body exercises like Wall Squats, Calf Raises, Side Leg Raises, and Wall Sits offer support and stability, making them accessible for all fitness levels. Integrating these exercises into a regular routine can contribute to enhanced posture, reduced injury risks, and increased confidence in daily activities.

The combined movements discussed, such as Wall Pilates Roll Down, Wall Leg Lifts with Arm Extensions, Lateral Wall Lunges with Reach, and Wall Supported Planks, highlight the importance of engaging multiple muscle groups simultaneously. These full-body exercises not only save time but also mimic everyday actions, promoting functional fitness. The adaptability of Wall Pilates ensures that seniors and beginners alike can benefit from these low-impact exercises, fostering better muscle coordination and overall agility. By committing to a consistent practice, individuals can achieve improved strength, flexibility, and balance, enhancing their quality of life.

All of this will lead us seamlessly into the next chapter, where we will delve into dynamic stretching techniques that not only prepare your body for exercise but also enhance overall performance and stability.

Chapter 4
Enhancing Flexibility and Balance

E nhancing flexibility and balance is integral to maintaining physical independence, especially as we age or begin new fitness routines. By focusing on these important elements through specialized Wall Pilates routines, this chapter aims to demonstrate their critical role in reducing the risk of injury and improving overall physical well-being. Flexibility allows for a greater range of motion in our joints, while balance helps us stay steady and coordinated, ensuring we can perform daily activities safely and efficiently.

Improved flexibility and balance also play a significant role in enhancing our athletic performance. Activities such as running, cycling, and dancing require a finely tuned body that can move quickly and with precision. When we increase our flexibility, our muscles can stretch more easily, which can lead to better strides in running or more fluid movements in dance. Balance ensures we do not falter or lose our footing, especially during quick changes in direction. This can prevent falls and maintain our speed and efficiency in a variety of sports.

With better flexibility and balance, engaging in recreational hobbies becomes more enjoyable and less risky. Whether it's playing a game of basketball or going for a hike, individuals with these skills can navigate uneven ground, jump, or pivot without worry. The joy of being active can be overshadowed by the fear of injury, but enhancing these physical attributes builds confidence. People can feel more comfortable trying new activities or pushing their limits, knowing their body can keep up.

Having good balance and flexibility also contributes to better posture. Poor posture can lead to discomfort and pain, especially for those who spend hours working at a desk or using electronic devices. Stretching and maintaining flexibility in the back, neck, and shoulders can help alleviate tension. Improved balance aids in standing tall and aligned, ensuring our bodies are in harmony. With better posture, we can breathe easier, reducing fatigue and creating a sense of well-being.

These attributes also enhance our mental health and relaxation. Movement practices that emphasize flexibility and balance, like yoga or Pilates, often incorporate mindful breathing and meditation. This combination not only improves physical abilities but also lowers stress levels and enhances our ability to focus. By practicing these elements regularly, individuals may find an increase in their overall mood and mental clarity, contributing to a more balanced life outside of physical activity.

Improved flexibility and balance are also beneficial for our daily routines. Simple tasks like reaching for an item on a shelf, bending down to tie shoelaces, or getting in and out of a car become effortless with increased muscle elasticity and body awareness. Everyday movements that once felt challenging become seamless, leading to a higher quality of life. Taking care of small chores around the house can feel less like a burden and more like an enjoyable activity.

As we continue to hone our flexibility and balance, we empower ourselves to remain active and engaged, fostering a lifestyle that embraces movement and exploration. It opens the door to social interactions, as participating in group activities, classes, or sports becomes more appealing. Engaging with our community while pursuing these activities can create lasting bonds and friendships, enriching our lives further.

Investing time in enhancing flexibility and balance is an investment in overall health and happiness. It provides a foundation for a vibrant and fulfilling life where movement is celebrated, not feared. As we prioritize these skills, we unlock a world filled with opportunities for fun, connection, and a deeper appreciation for our body's capabilities. The journey is rewarding, and the benefits ripple out into other areas of our lives, creating a more holistic approach to well-being.

Dynamic Stretching Techniques

Dynamic stretching plays a crucial role in Wall Pilates, especially when it comes to preparing your body for physical activity. These stretches involve moving parts of your body through their full range of motion. This can help in warming up your muscles and increasing your heart rate. For instance, if you are planning to engage in leg workouts, performing leg swings before you start can elevate your body temperature and make your muscles more pliable.

The benefits of dynamic stretching extend beyond just warming up. When you engage in these movements, you promote blood flow not just to your muscles but also to your joints. Better blood circulation means your muscles receive more oxygen, which is essential for optimal performance. When the muscles are well-nourished with oxygen and nutrients, they can work more efficiently, helping you achieve better results in your Pilates session.

Incorporating dynamic stretches specifically increases your range of motion. This is particularly important in Wall Pilates, where flexibility can determine the effectiveness of each exercise. For example, if you do not stretch your hamstrings before starting a session, you might find it hard to perform moves that require you to extend your legs fully. Dynamic stretching can help you attain a better range of motion, allowing for deeper stretches and more effective workouts.

When you focus on exercises that increase your flexibility, you also prepare yourself to prevent injuries. Tight muscles are more prone to strains and pulls. By continually performing dynamic stretches, you are actively working on lengthening your muscles. This is beneficial not only for Pilates but also for everyday activities.

Being mindful of how you execute dynamic stretches can be equally as important as the stretches themselves. Always move through your stretches smoothly and avoid jerky movements that can cause injury. Listen to your body; if a particular movement feels too intense, ease up. The aim is to prepare your body, not to overexert yourself before your Pilates session begins.

To effectively incorporate dynamic stretching into your routine, start with small movements that engage different muscle groups. A good step is to establish a warm-up period before your workout. Set aside about 5 to 10 minutes for dynamic stretching.

Warm-up

Warm-up movements play a crucial role in readying the body for physical activity. They are designed to elevate your heart rate, boost circulation, and warm up the muscles, thereby minimizing the risk of strains or sprains. One effective warm-up exercise involves standing with your feet shoulder-width apart, arms relaxed by your sides. Begin by slowly raising your arms above your head while inhaling deeply. Hold this position for a few seconds, then lower your arms while exhaling. Repeat this movement five times to enhance blood flow and oxygen delivery to your muscles.

Neck and Shoulder Rolls

Neck and shoulder rolls are essential techniques for releasing tension in the upper body, particularly beneficial for those who spend prolonged periods sitting at a desk.

Neck Rolls

To perform neck rolls, stand with your back against the wall, feet hip-width apart. Gently tilt your head to one side, bringing your ear toward your shoulder without lifting your shoulder. Slowly roll your head forward and down, tracing an imaginary half-circle with your chin until your other ear approaches the opposite shoulder. Roll your head back to the starting position and repeat three times on each side to help loosen tight neck muscles.

Shoulder Rolls

For shoulder rolls, maintain the same stance. Inhale deeply and lift your shoulders toward your ears. With a smooth, controlled motion, move them backward, squeezing your shoulder blades together, then exhale as you lower your shoulders. Continue rolling your shoulders forward, completing the circle. Perform ten slow, deliberate rolls in each direction to effectively reduce upper body tension and promote relaxation (Lindberg, 2020).

Hip Openers

Hip openers are another dynamic stretch vital for maintaining hip flexibility, and crucial for performing daily activities such as walking, bending, and lifting. Start by standing about a foot away from the wall, facing it. Place your hands flat on the wall at shoulder height for support. Lift your right knee to hip level and rotate your leg outward, opening the hip joint. This movement should form a circular motion akin to drawing half a circle with your knee. Perform ten circles clockwise and then counterclockwise before switching to the left leg. This exercise helps to lubricate the hip joints, improve mobility, and prevent stiffness (Burgess, 2019).

Leg Swings

Leg swings are highly effective dynamic stretches that target the muscles of the legs, hips, and lower back. They are performed using the wall for stability and come in two variations: lateral and forward leg swings.

Lateral

To do lateral leg swings, stand sideways to the wall with one hand resting on it for balance. Swing your outside leg gently across your body's midline and then out to the side. Aim for a controlled, rhythmic movement, repeating the swing ten times. Switch sides to work both legs equally.

Forward

Forward leg swings require you to face the wall, with both hands placed on it at shoulder height. Stand tall and swing one leg forward and backward in a smooth, continuous motion. Focus on keeping your torso upright and engaging your core muscles. Do ten forward swings with each leg, ensuring a full range of motion. These swings help activate the hip flexors, hamstrings, and glutes, preparing them for more intense activities.

Incorporating these dynamic stretching methods into your Wall Pilates routine can lead to remarkable improvements in flexibility and overall physical well-being. By diligently practicing these dynamic stretches, you create a strong foundation for successful Wall Pilates sessions. They ensure that your body is adequately prepared for exercise, allowing you to maximize the benefits of each workout while minimizing the potential for strain or injury. These stretches are invaluable tools for enhancing flexibility and promoting overall physical health.

By integrating these practices into your Wall Pilates routine, you stand a better chance of enjoying a fulfilling workout experience. With improved range of motion and reduced risk of injury, you can focus on achieving your fitness goals rather than worrying about how your body may react during the workout. This structured approach will inevitably lead to better performance, ensuring that you make the most of every session.

Balance-Focused Exercises

Enhancing balance through specific Wall Pilates exercises offers a gateway to stability and coordination, particularly beneficial for those seeking low-impact routines. Utilizing the wall as a support system can be an invaluable tool in these exercises, providing the necessary assistance while challenging balance capabilities.

Wall Pilates can improve balance by enhancing core strength. A strong core provides stability to the entire body. As individuals engage in exercises that activate their abdominal muscles, they learn to control their movements better. Techniques such as wall roll downs or the wall leg lifts require keeping the core engaged while using the wall for support. This creates a focus on maintaining a solid center, which translates into better balance in daily activities.

Incorporating dynamic movements into wall workouts can also be beneficial. By performing exercises that involve reaching, bending, or twisting while maintaining contact with the wall, individuals can challenge their balance further. This helps the body adapt to shifting weight and encourages quicker reactions to balance shifts. These dynamic actions foster agility, which is crucial for improving overall balance.

Breathing techniques also play a role in balance improvement. Practicing controlled breathing during exercises brings awareness to body alignment and helps individuals stay grounded. Deep, focused breaths can calm the mind, improving concentration during complex movements. When the mind is clear, it becomes easier to feel the body's balance and alignment. This connection between breath and body in wall Pilates enhances the practitioner's ability to maintain steadiness.

Single-Leg Stand

One effective exercise to enhance balance and core engagement is the Single-Leg Stand. This exercise uses the wall to assist in maintaining stability while focusing on standing on one leg. To perform the Single-Leg Stand, position yourself near a wall with your side almost touching it. Slowly lift one foot off the ground, engaging your core muscles to keep your body upright. The wall provides a supportive structure, helping you maintain balance as you hold the position for several seconds. Repeat this exercise on both legs, gradually increasing the duration as your balance improves. This drill not only strengthens the core but also enhances proprioception, the body's ability to sense its position and movement, which is crucial for overall stability.

Wall Squats

Wall Squats are another integral exercise that targets strength and balance simultaneously. Begin by standing with your back against the wall, feet shoulder-width apart and slightly away from the wall. Slowly lower yourself into a squat position, ensuring your knees don't extend past your toes. Maintain contact between your back and the wall throughout the movement. This controlled exercise builds lower body strength, particularly in the quadriceps and glutes, while also engaging the core muscles for stabilization. By using the wall, you can safely challenge your balance and gradually improve your squat depth as you gain confidence and strength. Wall Squats provide a stable method to address balance challenges, especially for beginners or those with limited mobility.

Heel-to-Toe Walk

Practicing the Heel-to-Toe Walk along a wall is a straightforward yet effective way to improve stability. For this exercise, start by positioning yourself next to a wall with one hand lightly touching it for support. Place the heel of one foot directly in front of the toes of the other foot, creating a straight line. Walk forward slowly, maintaining this heel-to-toe alignment. Focus on moving with control and stability, using the wall for balance if needed. This simple exercise mimics natural walking patterns while emphasizing deliberate, balanced steps. It helps reinforce proper gait mechanics and enhances overall stability, making everyday activities safer and more manageable.

Lateral Leg Lifts

Lateral Leg Lifts incorporate the wall as a support tool to focus on lateral stability. Stand beside the wall with your hand resting lightly against it for balance. Lift your outside leg to the side, keeping it straight and engaging your core muscles throughout the movement. Hold the position briefly before lowering your leg back down. Perform multiple repetitions on each side, gradually increasing the number as your balance and lateral strength improve. This exercise targets the muscles on the sides of the hips and thighs, essential for stabilizing the pelvis and improving side-to-side balance. Lateral Leg Lifts play a significant role in enhancing functional movements, such as stepping sideways or adjusting balance during unexpected shifts in weight.

Gentle Stretching Routines for Seniors

Enhancing flexibility and mobility is crucial for seniors to maintain their independence and reduce the risk of injuries. One effective way to achieve this is through carefully designed stretching routines that can be performed safely, even from a seated position. These stretches not only help in improving the range of motion but also ensure that the exercises are gentle on the body while providing significant benefits.

Stretching is essential for seniors because it helps maintain joint health. As people age, joints can become stiff, leading to discomfort and decreased mobility. Stretching keeps the body flexible and can ease tension in the muscles. This is particularly important for seniors who may have arthritis or other conditions that affect their joints. By incorporating gentle stretches into their daily routine, seniors can reduce pain and increase their ability to move comfortably.

Regular stretching can also improve circulation. Good blood flow is vital for overall health and energy levels. When seniors stretch, they encourage blood flow to their muscles and joints, delivering oxygen and nutrients that promote healing and vitality. Improved circulation can help seniors feel more energized and less fatigued throughout the day. As they become more active, they may find that everyday tasks are easier to perform, boosting their confidence and encouraging them to stay engaged in activities they enjoy.

Many falls among seniors result from balance issues, which can be exacerbated by tight muscles and limited mobility. Stretching enhances balance by increasing body awareness and coordination. When seniors focus on their posture and alignment during stretching, they also strengthen their ability to maintain stability. This can be particularly helpful in preventing falls at home or while out and about. A simple stretching routine can make a significant difference, allowing seniors to navigate their environment more safely.

Many seniors experience aches and pains that can interfere with their enjoyment of life. Stretching serves as a natural pain relief method, helping to ease muscle tightness and promote relaxation. When seniors take the time to stretch, they often find relief from discomfort associated with back pain, stiffness, and tension headaches. This simple act can foster a greater sense of calm and reduce the risk of developing more serious conditions related to chronic pain. Regular stretching sessions provide a few quiet moments to unwind and care for oneself, which is invaluable for mental health.

Stretching can lead to improved sleep quality. Many seniors struggle with sleep issues, which can be exacerbated by physical discomfort and anxiety. Gentle stretching exercises before bedtime can relax muscles and calm the mind, making it easier to drift off. By establishing a nightly routine that includes stretching, seniors can promote deeper, more restorative sleep. When they wake up feeling refreshed, they are more likely to approach the day with a positive attitude and a willingness to participate in activities that foster their independence.

Staying proactive about physical health is essential for seniors, and stretching is an excellent way to take charge of their wellbeing. It empowers seniors to make choices that enhance their mobility and overall quality of life. As they notice improvements in their ability to move, they also become more motivated to keep up with their routines. Simple exercises, whether done alone or in a group setting, can reignite a sense of purpose and enjoyment in daily activities.

As seniors embark on their stretching journey, it's important to listen to their bodies and not push themselves too hard. Every body is different, and what feels good for one person may not feel good for another. A focus on gradual progression is key, celebrating the small victories along the way. Feeling the benefits of stretching builds confidence and makes it easier to stick with it over time. Before long, stretching will become an enjoyable and rewarding part of their daily lives, enhancing both physical and emotional health.

Seated Wall Stretch

The Seated Wall Stretch is an ideal starting point. This stretch can be performed while seated, making it safe and accessible for those who may have difficulties standing. Begin by sitting comfortably on a chair placed near a wall. Ensure your back is straight and feet flat on the floor. Raise your arms above your head, then gently lean forward towards the wall without rounding your lower back. Hold this position for 10 to 30 seconds, feeling a mild stretch in your hamstrings and lower back. Repeat as necessary. This simple movement helps loosen tight muscles and enhances flexibility, preparing you for more dynamic activities throughout the day.

Side Body Stretch

Next, the Side Body Stretch targets the lateral muscles along the side of your torso, which often become stiff with age. Stand or sit beside a wall with your legs shoulder-width apart. Raise your left arm overhead and place your right hand on the wall for support. Slowly lean to the right, feeling the stretch along the left side of your body. Hold the stretch for 10 to 30 seconds, then return to the starting position and switch sides. By using the wall for support, you maintain balance and stability, ensuring the exercise is performed safely. This routine not only increases flexibility but also helps in maintaining proper posture.

Calf Stretch Against the Wall

Calf stretches are essential for maintaining lower leg flexibility, which can affect overall mobility. The Calf Stretch Against the Wall is an effective way to focus on these muscles. Position yourself facing a wall, placing both hands against it at shoulder height. Step one foot back, keeping it straight, while bending the front knee slightly. Press your back heel into the ground until you feel a stretch in your calf. Hold for 10 to 30 seconds before switching legs. For additional support, you can modify this by performing it seated in a chair, extending one leg out, and gently pulling your toes towards you. Regularly practicing this stretch can help alleviate stiffness and prevent cramps, contributing to better walking stability.

Upper Back Stretch

Stretches targeting the upper spine are vital for enhancing mobility and relieving tension in the back muscles. To perform the Upper Back Stretch, stand or sit with your feet shoulder-width apart, facing a wall. Raise your arms and place your palms against the wall at shoulder height. Engage your core and slowly push your chest towards the wall, feeling a gentle stretch in your upper back and shoulders. Maintain this position for 10 to 30 seconds, breathing deeply throughout. This stretch can help reduce discomfort caused by prolonged periods of sitting or screen time, promoting better spinal health and posture.

Guidelines for Safe Stretching

When performing any stretching routine, it's essential to follow some fundamental guidelines to maximize safety and effectiveness. Always warm up before stretching by walking in place for a few minutes to get your blood flowing and muscles warm. Focus on deep, steady breathing and listen to your body to avoid pushing too far. If any movement causes pain, stop immediately and consider consulting a healthcare professional. It's also advisable to use modifications, such as performing stretches while seated or using supports like walls and chairs to enhance stability.

Maximizing Benefits and Maintaining Routine

Creating a consistent stretching routine can significantly improve flexibility and mobility over time. Aim to incorporate these stretches daily, whether in the morning to start your day or in the evening to unwind. Consistency helps in building muscle memory and gradually increases your range of motion. Engaging in regular exercises like walking or light pilates can complement these stretches and provide a balanced fitness regimen tailored to your needs.

Consistency in practice and progression is key to reaping the full benefits of these exercises. Start with shorter durations and fewer repetitions, gradually increasing as you become more comfortable and confident. It's also important to listen to your body and avoid pushing beyond your limits, ensuring a safe and effective routine.

Beyond individual exercises, integrating these movements into a regular fitness regimen promotes overall physical independence and reduces the risk of falls and injuries. As highlighted by Healthline, "Improving balance increases coordination and strength, allowing you to move freely and steadily" (Cronkleton, 2019). This holistic approach not only makes daily tasks easier but also enhances athletic performance and mental focus, contributing to a well-rounded sense of wellness.

For seniors, the emphasis on balance exercises cannot be overstated. More than three million older Americans visit emergency rooms annually due to fall-related injuries, underscoring the critical need for preventative measures (Clinic, 2021). Engaging in these Wall Pilates exercises can significantly contribute to reducing such risks, promoting a safer and more active lifestyle. Incorporating these exercises into daily routines, even for just a few minutes, can make a substantial difference in maintaining physical health and independence.

Addressing Common Flexibility Challenges

Addressing common flexibility challenges is a matter of understanding and adapting to one's body limitations. Flexibility plays a vital role in both maintaining overall physical health and enhancing the quality of movement. For both seniors and beginners, recognizing the areas where tightness occurs is crucial for progressing in any fitness journey. Awareness and proactive measures can prevent injuries and lead to a more enjoyable exercise experience. Recognizing this need, we delve into identifying these specific regions of tightness and offer practical strategies to address them.

Identifying Tight Areas

When embarking on a fitness journey, one of the fundamental aspects to consider is flexibility. Flexibility plays a crucial role in maintaining functional strength, enhancing balance, and improving overall movement quality. To effectively enhance flexibility, it is essential to educate readers on recognizing common tightness regions within their bodies. This section aims to foster an understanding that awareness of these tight areas can significantly aid in self-care, prevention of injuries, and a more enjoyable practice experience.

Awareness of one's body limitations is the first step towards fostering self-care and prevention. When individuals are conscious of which parts of their body tend to tighten, they are better equipped to take precautions during physical activities. For instance, seniors often experience tightness in areas such as the lower back, hamstrings, and hip flexors, primarily due to prolonged sitting or reduced physical activity. By recognizing these tight regions, they can integrate specific stretches aimed at loosening these muscles into their routine, thereby reducing the risk of strains and other related injuries.

For beginners, acknowledging their body's limitations helps prevent overexertion, which could potentially lead to injuries. An informed approach to stretching allows them to listen to their bodies and recognize when to stop pushing further. This mindful engagement not only fosters safe practice but also builds a foundation for a sustainable fitness journey. Practicing mindfulness in stretching encourages individuals to appreciate the process rather than rush through exercises, ultimately leading to incremental yet significant improvements in flexibility.

Being proactive about flexibility improvement is another critical aspect of addressing common tightness regions. When individuals actively seek to understand and improve their tightness areas, they adopt a more engaged approach to their fitness routines. Instead of passively performing stretches, they become participants in their well-being journey. This proactive stance can include incorporating different types of stretches targeted at tight areas. For example, if someone identifies that their calf muscles are particularly tight, they can perform calf raises, heel drops, and dynamic ankle circles as part of their warm-up routine. Dynamic stretching, prior to engaging in physical activity, prepares the muscles by moving joints through their full range of motion without holding a stretch. Such targeted actions can greatly enhance the effectiveness of their efforts in improving flexibility.

Understanding one's body limitations enhances the overall practice experience. When individuals are knowledgeable about their physical constraints, they can tailor their exercise routines to cater to their needs, thereby making each session more enjoyable and productive. This understanding fosters a positive relationship with their bodies, where the focus shifts from merely reaching flexibility goals to appreciating the progress made. For seniors, this might mean adapting certain exercises using modifications or props such as straps and blocks, allowing them to comfortably participate in activities like yoga or Pilates without feeling overwhelmed. For beginners, understanding their body's tight areas can help in setting realistic goals and celebrating small milestones, which is crucial in maintaining motivation.

Recognizing tight areas is pivotal in targeting specific stretches. Familiarity with these regions ensures that the stretches performed are not generic but rather tailored to address individual needs. Common tightness areas such as the lower back, shoulders, neck, hamstrings, and calves can be addressed through specific stretches. For example, lower back tightness can be alleviated through gentle forward bends while seated or standing, ensuring the spine is elongated and not compressed. For the shoulders and neck, stretches such as shoulder rolls, neck tilts, and cross-body arm stretches can help release tension effectively. Hamstrings can benefit from leg raises or seated stretches, while calf muscles can be loosened with standing calf stretches or downward-facing dog pose in yoga.

Identifying specific tightness regions helps in creating a balanced stretching routine that addresses both prominent and subtle areas of tension. This balance prevents overemphasis on one area while neglecting others, promoting holistic flexibility improvement. It also helps in avoiding the common mistake of performing the same stretches repeatedly without addressing the actual areas of need. Regularly assessing and responding to the body's signals ensures that the flexibility regimen evolves with the individual's progress and changing needs.

Incorporating specific stretches based on recognized tightness not only improves flexibility but also enhances overall physical performance. For instance, improved hamstring flexibility can lead to better posture and reduced lower back pain, while flexible shoulders and neck can alleviate discomfort caused by long hours of sedentary work. Targeting these tight areas contributes to enhanced mobility, making daily activities such as bending, lifting, and walking more fluid and less strenuous.

Using the Wall for Support

Using wall support in flexibility exercises provides an accessible way for seniors and beginners to achieve effective stretches while preventing falls. Walls offer a sturdy prop, enabling individuals to maintain balance and reduce the risk of injury during their practice. Stretching can be intimidating, especially if you're worried about losing your footing or overextending yourself. The wall acts as a safety net, allowing users to focus on their movements without fear. For instance, when performing a hamstring stretch with one leg up against the wall, it becomes easier to gauge the depth of the stretch and control the intensity. This makes it more likely to perform the exercise correctly and get the intended benefit.

Wall support also helps increase the range of motion safely and gradually. By leaning into the wall for various stretches, you can extend your reach slowly and steadily without straining. Imagine trying to improve shoulder flexibility by doing wall slides; standing with your back against the wall and sliding your arms upward engages the shoulder muscles effectively. This incremental approach is crucial for seniors who might have joint issues or limited mobility. It ensures that they aren't pushing too hard too soon, which could lead to setbacks rather than improvements.

Practical adjustments to routines are another advantage of using wall support. Integrating wall exercises into your daily schedule can make stretching less daunting and more reachable. Mornings can begin with gentle wall stretches to jumpstart the day, while evenings may close with wall-assisted calf stretches to unwind. These subtle additions help build a consistent routine that is easy to stick with. When stretches are framed as part of everyday activities, like reaching up to change a light bulb or bending down to pick something off the floor, it becomes more natural to incorporate them consistently.

Mindful Engagement

Mindful engagement plays a significant role in enhancing the benefits of flexibility practices. While leveraging wall support, participants can cultivate a deeper connection between their mind and body. Mental focus techniques such as visualization and deep breathing can be incorporated seamlessly into the process. For example, envisioning each muscle group elongating during the stretch not only improves physical flexibility but also reinforces mental awareness. Mindfulness reduces the risk of overexertion by promoting attentiveness to bodily signals, ensuring exercises are performed within safe limits. Focused breathing techniques, akin to those used in Wall Pilates, enhance this connection, turning each stretch into a mini-meditation session that calms the mind while working the body (Hardy, 2024).

Encouraging a deeper connection through mindful engagement fosters patience in flexibility progress. Sometimes, the journey to becoming more flexible is slow, and it's easy to become discouraged. However, by practicing mindfulness, individuals learn to appreciate small gains and enjoy the process rather than just focusing on the end goal. This attitude can be particularly beneficial for seniors and beginners who might feel overwhelmed by the changes they need to make. By enjoying each step and acknowledging how their bodies respond to different stretches, they create a positive feedback loop that encourages continued practice.

Stretching Frequency

Regular stretching builds new habits that enhance muscle length and overall flexibility. Consistency is key in seeing tangible results. Making stretching a daily or near-daily habit ensures that muscles are continually being worked and expanded. Even short sessions, when done regularly, can lead to significant improvements over time. Consider integrating these sessions into your morning routine or evening wind-down; the regularity helps form lasting habits that contribute to long-term flexibility.

Incorporating stretches as part of daily activities further solidifies these habits. Simple actions like stretching your calves while brushing your teeth or doing shoulder rolls during TV commercials can seamlessly integrate into your day. These micro-sessions don't require dedicated workout time and thus feel less burdensome. Over weeks and months, these small efforts accumulate, leading to noticeable enhancements in flexibility without major lifestyle disruptions. Just like remembering to stay hydrated, integrating frequent, short stretches into mundane tasks ensures that the practice of flexibility becomes second nature.

Providing suggestions for practical scheduling to integrate flexibility work is essential. For those looking to establish a consistent routine, creating a straightforward schedule can make all the difference. Start with realistic goals—perhaps dedicating ten minutes each morning and evening. Utilize prompts like calendar reminders or apps specifically designed for tracking fitness progress. A weekly planner might include varied stretches targeting different muscle groups, ensuring a well-rounded approach. Monday could focus on hip stretches, Wednesday on upper body flexibility, and Friday on lower body stretches. Such structure prevents monotony and keeps the practice engaging.

A suggested practical schedule for beginners might look like this:

Monday:

Morning: Wall-Assisted Hamstring Stretches

Evening: Calf Stretches against the Wall

Wednesday:

Morning: Wall Slides for Shoulder Flexibility

Evening: Wall Push-ups to engage the upper body

Friday:

Morning: Wall Squats to strengthen lower body muscles

Evening: Gentle Wall Planks to activate core stability

By creating a balanced and varied schedule, individuals ensure that they target multiple areas without overwhelming themselves with too many tasks at once. This format also allows for adequate recovery time, which is vital in any exercise regimen, particularly for seniors or those new to fitness routines.

Leveraging tools like wall support can make stretching exercises more accessible and safer, encouraging consistency without the fear of overexertion. Creating practical schedules and incorporating stretches into daily activities were highlighted as effective strategies to build lasting habits and achieve holistic physical well-being. This reflective approach to flexibility allows both seniors and beginners to appreciate their progress and maintain motivation, ultimately leading to a more enjoyable and beneficial fitness journey.

Embracing the Lessons Learned

The structured support provided by the wall allows for modifications and adjustments tailored to individual needs. Whether you're a senior aiming to preserve functional strength or a beginner seeking a gentle introduction to fitness, these exercises offer adaptable solutions. The simplicity and effectiveness of using a wall for support align well with the diverse abilities and requirements of individuals across different age groups.

We have explored various techniques aimed at enhancing flexibility and balance through Wall Pilates routines. By incorporating dynamic stretching methods, individuals can significantly improve their range of motion and reduce the risk of injuries. These exercises prepare the body effectively for physical activity, ensuring that participants can perform more intensive workouts safely and with greater ease.

As we conclude our exploration of targeted Wall Pilates exercises, it's essential to recognize that the effectiveness of these movements extends beyond physical strength. In the next chapter, we will delve into the vital role of breathing, emphasizing how mastering diaphragmatic breathing can significantly enhance relaxation, focus, and overall performance.

Chapter 5
Mindfulness Practices in Wall Pilates

Integrating mindfulness into Wall Pilates fosters a deeper connection between the body and mind, promoting both physical health and mental well-being. Far from being mere physical exercises, mindful practices transform Wall Pilates into holistic experiences that nurture one's entire being. This chapter delves into the various techniques and strategies for embedding mindfulness into your Wall Pilates routine, aiming to elevate your workout beyond simple mechanical movements.

Approaching daily situations with a mindful mindset allows for greater patience and clarity. Whether dealing with a stressful work environment or navigating personal relationships, the principles of mindfulness learned in Wall Pilates can provide a foundation for more thoughtful responses. Practitioners often report increased self-awareness, emotional balance, and overall appreciation for life. These practices cultivate resilience, helping individuals better navigate challenges with grace. As the mind and body become more attuned, everyday experiences gain depth and meaning, enhancing the overall quality of life.

By allowing mindfulness to permeate Wall Pilates routines and daily activities, individuals set the foundation for lifelong practices that promote health, happiness, and harmony. The journey is not just about improving physical fitness but also about embracing a fuller, more enriching life experience. This holistic approach nurtures not only the individual but also the larger community as a whole, inspiring others to explore the transformative power of mindfulness.

Understanding the link between physical exercises and mental focus is important. Wall Pilates, by design, requires practitioners to engage deeply with each movement, ensuring precision and control. This attentiveness naturally demands concentration, which trains the mind to be present in the moment. As participants focus on their alignment and movements, they inherently develop better mental clarity and enhanced cognitive function (Hardy, 2024). The deliberate movements in Wall Pilates necessitate an acute awareness of one's body, fostering a mind-body connection that extends beyond the practice itself. For both seniors looking to maintain functional strength and younger fitness enthusiasts seeking consistency, this heightened mental engagement can lead to noticeable improvements in overall mindfulness and stress management.

Breathwork is another pivotal component of Wall Pilates that integrates mindfulness into physical exercise. Proper breathing techniques are essential for executing Pilates exercises effectively. In Wall Pilates, breath control is not just about oxygen intake; it's a fundamental part of the practice that supports muscle engagement and relaxation. Practitioners are encouraged to inhale deeply through the nose and exhale fully through the mouth, synchronizing breaths with movements. This controlled breathing pattern helps regulate the nervous system, reduce stress levels, and enhance mental clarity (Cleveland Clinic, 2023). By focusing on breathwork, practitioners learn to calm their minds and remain present, which is particularly beneficial for older adults who may experience anxiety or stress.

Being present and aware within one's experience is a core principle of Wall Pilates. Unlike high-intensity workouts where speed and repetition are prioritized, Wall Pilates encourages slow, deliberate movements that require full attention. This approach not only minimizes the risk of injury but also maximizes the benefits of each exercise. Practitioners are guided to pay close attention to how their bodies feel during each movement, noticing any areas of tension or discomfort. This mindfulness helps individuals understand their physical limits and capabilities, promoting a sense of self-awareness and body confidence.

Wall Pilates offers numerous benefits, not only for physical fitness but also for mental focus and mindfulness. This section will delve into the mindful aspects of Wall Pilates, emphasizing how the practice cultivates a strong connection between physical exercises and mental clarity.

Breathing Techniques for Relaxation

Breathing is the cornerstone of a mindful Wall Pilates practice, serving as a bridge between physical exercise and mental relaxation. This section explores effective breathing methods to enhance relaxation and focus during Wall Pilates exercises. Understanding how to harness your breath can elevate your practice, making it more beneficial for both mind and body.

Breathing directly affects our nervous system. When we breathe deeply, it sends signals to our body to relax. A calm body leads to a calm mind. In Wall Pilates, this connection is crucial. It allows us to move through the exercises with purpose and intention. Focusing on our breath can also help us to become aware of any tension in our bodies. By paying attention to our breathing patterns, we can identify areas that may need more relaxation or relief. This awareness is the first step in fostering a more mindful practice.

The timing of our breaths matters too. Inhale deeply when preparing for a movement enhances stability. As we exhale, we release tension and create space for our bodies to move more freely. For example, when performing a wall roll-down, inhaling helps to lengthen the spine, while exhaling allows for a soft bending of the knees and a gentle forward fold. This cycle of breath keeps the flow steady and makes each movement more graceful. Practicing this rhythm transforms not just how we execute the exercises, but also how we feel throughout the session.

Another essential aspect of breathing in Wall Pilates lies in its role in energy management. Short, rapid breaths can lead to a feeling of unease and fatigue. On the other hand, slow, controlled breaths can help maintain energy levels and sustain endurance. This balance is vital, especially during more challenging sequences. When we feel ourselves struggling during a tough exercise, returning to our breath can center us. A few deep inhales and exhales can recharge our focus, allowing us to push through with resilience.

Incorporating breathing techniques into each exercise promotes a deeper sense of connection to our bodies. For example, during the 'Wall Push-Up,' inhaling as we lower and exhaling as we push away helps to synchronize our movements. This synchronization transforms the exercise into a flowing dance rather than rigid reps. Feel the rhythm of breathing guiding each action. Over time, this connection enhances muscle memory, making the practice feel more intuitive and fulfilling.

It's also helpful to explore different breathing patterns. Some practitioners prefer breathing through the nose for a more calming effect, while others might find that exhaling through the mouth better suits their practice. Experiment with both techniques during your workouts to discover which feels more natural. The beauty of Wall Pilates is that it can be tailored to individual needs. Our breath is the thread that weaves personal preference into our routines.

Integrating breath work with intention also prepares us for transitions in our practice. This is especially evident in movements that require a shift in energy or focus. When moving from a more intense cardio-inspired sequence to a gentle stretch, guiding our breath alongside these transitions can ease the shift. Allow a few moments of deep breathing before starting the new phase. This moment helps to reset the mind and body, signaling it's time to embrace a different pace and energy.

Understanding the anatomy of breath can further deepen the practice. Awareness of the diaphragm's role in breathing can enhance our ability to create space in the torso during movement. As we engage the diaphragm with each inhale, the ribs expand and the lungs fill, providing essential oxygen. This improved exchange not only boosts our energy but also nurtures a sense of well-being. Focusing on the mechanics of breathing can turn a simple task into a powerful tool for support in Wall Pilates.

Mindfulness extends beyond the mat. When we bring conscious breathing into our daily lives, we carry its benefits everywhere. Simple awareness of breath during stressful moments can help center us. Entering a crowded space or facing a challenging conversation, pausing to take a few deep breaths can bring clarity and calm. This practice teaches us that mindfulness is not confined to our workout sessions, but rather a lifestyle.

With these strategies rooted in our practice, nurturing relaxation and focus becomes a seamless part of our Wall Pilates journey. Finding moments of stillness amidst the movement solidifies our commitment to health, both physically and mentally. Each deep breath reinforces our purpose and motivation for practicing. It's about more than just exercise; it's a holistic approach to well-being. Inviting breath into each segment creates an experience that resonates far beyond the wall.

As we journey deeper, incorporating mindfulness and breath awareness can profoundly enhance our connection with ourselves and our surroundings. Embrace this opportunity to explore the subtleties of each breath. Notice how it influences your posture, energy, and mindset. In time, this practice can lead us to discover the remarkable resilience and strength that lies within. Finding joy in each breath further enriches the Wall Pilates experience, laying the groundwork for continuous growth and self-awareness.

Diaphragmatic Breathing

Understanding diaphragmatic breathing is crucial for any Pilates practice. This foundational technique involves deep abdominal breathing, which promotes full oxygen exchange in the lungs. By focusing on expanding the diaphragm rather than just the chest, you ensure that your body receives ample oxygen, which calms the nervous system and enhances concentration. More oxygen not only fuels your muscles but also sharpens your mental clarity, allowing you to stay present and engaged in your exercises. Diaphragmatic breathing supports this by fostering a state of relaxation and reducing stress, essential for anyone looking to balance their physical fitness with mental well-being.

One way to practice diaphragmatic breathing is by lying on your back with one hand on your chest and the other on your abdomen. As you inhale deeply through your nose, aim to raise the hand on your abdomen while keeping the hand on your chest relatively still. This helps you ensure that the diaphragm, not the chest, is doing most of the work. As you exhale slowly through your mouth, allow your abdomen to fall. This simple exercise can be done anywhere and serves as a great introduction to efficient breathing techniques, encouraging a habit of mindful inhalation and exhalation.

Breath Coordination with Movement

Synchronizing your breath with your movements can enhance physical awareness and significantly reduce the risk of injury. When you align your breath with your Pilates exercises, you create a harmonious flow that amplifies each movement's effectiveness. For instance, inhaling during the preparation phase of a movement fills the body with energy, while exhaling during exertion helps stabilize the core and control the motion. This intentional coupling of breath and movement ensures that muscles are adequately oxygenated when they are working hardest, thereby enhancing performance and preventing unnecessary strain.

To practice breath coordination, begin with a basic Wall Pilates exercise like the wall roll-down. Stand with your back against the wall, feet hip-distance apart, arms relaxed by your sides. Inhale deeply, feeling your rib cage expand, and then, as you exhale, slowly roll down vertebra by vertebra until your hands reach your knees or shins. Pause, take a deep breath in, and then exhale as you roll back up. This exercise synchronizes breath with movement, promoting better physical alignment and increasing body awareness.

Visualization with Breath

Visualization with breath adds another layer to your Wall Pilates practice, encouraging mental engagement and a positive mindset. Visualization techniques involve imagining the air you inhale filling different parts of your body with light or energy, and visualizing tension leaving your body with each exhale. This not only aids in physical relaxation but also cultivates a sense of mindfulness, helping you stay focused and motivated throughout your session. Visualization can transform routine exercises into a more immersive experience, where the mind actively participates in the body's movements.

A practical example of visualization with breath can be found in the "wall bridge" exercise. Lie on your back with your feet pressed against the wall, knees bent at a 90-degree angle. As you inhale, visualize your breath traveling down to your pelvis, filling it with warmth and light. On the exhale, imagine this light extending through your legs and out through your toes, releasing any tension. This mental imagery reinforces physical relaxation and strengthens the connection between mind and body.

Breath-Focused Exercises

Practicing breath-focused exercises regularly can help embed these beneficial habits into your daily routine. Simple routines designed to enhance breath awareness can lay the foundation for lasting change, turning conscious breathing into an automatic response during your workouts. Consistency is key here; dedicate a few minutes each day to practice these techniques to build a strong, resilient breathing pattern.

One such breath-focused exercise involves standing against the wall with your feet hip-width apart. Place your hands on your lower ribs. Inhale deeply through your nose, feeling your ribs expand sideways. Hold the breath for a moment, then exhale slowly through pursed lips, feeling your ribs contract. Repeat this process several times, each time trying to deepen the inhalation and lengthen the exhalation. This routine not only improves breath control but also engages the core muscles, making it an effective dual-purpose exercise.

Mindful Movement Sequences

Engaging in mindful movement sequences during Wall Pilates can enhance your overall workout experience by fostering a deeper connection and heightened awareness of both body and mind. This section aims to guide you through the process of incorporating mindfulness into your Wall Pilates practice, ensuring every movement is intentional and meaningful.

Slow and Intentional Movements

One fundamental aspect of mindful movement is slowing down and making each motion deliberate. Slow and intentional movements are essential for several reasons. Firstly, they promote safety. When you move slowly, you reduce the risk of injuries typically caused by hurried or careless motions. This is particularly important for seniors who may be more prone to falls and strains.

Secondly, slow movements have a meditative aspect. By focusing on each part of the movement, you turn your exercise session into a form of moving meditation. This can help calm the mind, reduce stress, and create a sense of inner peace. For example, when performing a wall sit, focus on feeling the pressure between your back and the wall, how your quadriceps engage, and ensure your knees stay aligned with your ankles.

Thirdly, there are sensory benefits to sloweddown exercises. Moving slowly allows you to tune into the sensations in your muscles and joints and become more aware of how your body responds to different positions. This heightened sensory awareness can deepen your understanding of your physical capabilities and limitations, facilitating better self-care in your exercise routine.

Body Awareness Practices

To further enhance your connection during Wall Pilates, incorporating body awareness practices like body scans and alignment cues is beneficial. A body scan involves mentally checking in with various parts of your body, starting from your toes and moving up to your head. This practice encourages mindfulness by directing your attention inward, allowing you to notice areas of tension, discomfort, or ease.

For instance, before beginning your Wall Pilates routine, take a few minutes to perform a body scan. Stand with your back against the wall and close your eyes. Slowly bring your awareness to your feet, noting any sensations without judgment. Gradually move your attention upwards, through your legs, torso, arms, and finally your head. This practice not only promotes relaxation but also helps you identify areas that might need extra care during your workout.

Alignment cues are another essential component of body awareness. These cues guide you in maintaining proper posture and technique, which is crucial for effective and safe workouts. For example, when performing a leg lift against the wall, an alignment cue might be to keep your pelvis neutral and avoid arching your lower back. Such cues ensure that you engage the correct muscles and prevent unnecessary strain.

Flowing Sequences

Creating smooth transitions between movements is another key element of mindful Wall Pilates. Flowing sequences help promote relaxation and reduce tension, making your workout more enjoyable and less taxing on your body. The idea is to maintain a continuous flow of movement rather than treating each exercise as a separate entity.

For example, you can transition from a wall sit into a leg lift by slowly shifting your weight onto one leg while lifting the other. Maintain a steady breath and focus on the fluidity of the transition. This approach encourages a sense of harmony and coherence in your practice, enhancing the overall mindfulness of the workout.

Flowing sequences also prevent the buildup of lactic acid in your muscles, reducing post-workout soreness. By keeping your movements smooth and connected, you sustain muscle engagement without overwhelming specific groups, fostering balanced strength and flexibility.

Feedback Tools

Incorporating feedback tools such as guided journals and prompts for self-reflection can significantly enhance your mindful Wall Pilates practice. Keeping a journal allows you to track your progress, set goals, and reflect on your experiences. This process not only provides valuable insights into your physical and mental growth but also keeps you motivated and engaged.

Start by documenting each session, noting down the exercises performed, duration, and any observations about your physical and emotional state. For example, you might write about how a particular exercise felt, any difficulties encountered, or moments of breakthrough and ease. Over time, this record becomes a powerful tool for self-assessment and improvement.

Prompts for self-reflection can include questions like, "How did I feel before and after the workout?" or "What was my level of focus during each movement?" Reflecting on these prompts helps you recognize patterns, celebrate progress, and address challenges. It fosters a deeper connection to your practice, reinforcing the importance of mindfulness in your Wall Pilates journey.

Consider seeking feedback from a certified Pilates instructor if possible. Regular check-ins with an expert can provide you with professional insights and corrections that are tailored to your individual needs. An instructor can offer valuable guidance on improving technique, adjusting exercises to suit your capabilities, and overcoming specific challenges.

Integrating mindfulness into your Wall Pilates practice transforms a simple workout into a holistic experience that nurtures both body and mind. By focusing on slow and intentional movements, you ensure safety, tap into the meditative aspects of exercise, and enjoy the sensory benefits of being fully present. Body awareness practices, such as body scans and alignment cues, deepen your connection to your physical self and promote better posture and technique.

Connecting Body and Mind Through Pilates

Wall Pilates effectively bridges the physical and mental realms, fostering a profound mind-body connection. This practice underscores how mindful movement can enhance our overall well-being, making it an invaluable tool.

Mind-body connection is essential for achieving a balanced life. It allows us to tune into our feelings and understand our needs better. When we are aware of how our body feels while moving, we can identify stress or tension before it grows into something larger. This practice encourages us to listen to ourselves, promoting relaxation and clarity. Being in tune with our emotions also helps us respond to life's challenges with greater awareness.

Developing this connection through Wall Pilates offers practical benefits. It strengthens the core while keeping our attention focused on the present moment. Each movement builds strength and flexibility, which can translate to improved physical activities outside of class. A strong core supports good posture and balance. As we become more physically adept, our confidence can grow, encouraging us to explore new activities or environments without the fear of injury.

Engaging in mindful movement also fosters emotional resilience. When we approach each exercise with intention, we learn to let go of distractions. This focus can reduce anxiety and promote a calmer mindset. The rhythm of our breathing combined with the flow of movement creates a meditative state. Over time, this practice cultivates patience and self-acceptance, essential elements for personal growth and well-being.

Despite the challenges we face, this practice encourages optimism. By focusing on what our bodies are capable of, instead of limitations, we develop a growth mindset. We learn to appreciate small victories, fostering gratitude. Each session becomes a celebration of our progress, no matter how minor. This shift in perspective helps us navigate obstacles in a more graceful manner.

Listening to our bodies is a skill acquired over time. It requires patience and practice but ultimately leads to empowerment. When we understand our limits and strengths, it encourages a compassionate relationship with ourselves. We become our own advocates, making choices that align with our well-being. This understanding is critical for developing a sustainable practice, as it prevents burnout and injury.

Over time, our relationship with movement matures. What once may have felt like a chore transforms into a cherished practice. The body becomes a vessel of expression, capable of conveying emotions through movement. Each exercise reflects our growth, serving as both a physical and emotional release.

Exploring nuances in this practice reveals rich layers of meaning. Each person's journey will be different, shaped by individual experiences and challenges. The beauty of Wall Pilates lies in its adaptability, catering to diverse needs and goals. This inclusivity invites everyone to engage, fostering a welcoming environment for all.

As the practice deepens, we begin to see how interconnected our lives are. The kinesiology of movement influences our emotional landscape, while our thoughts affect our physical performance. Through this lens, the mind-body connection transforms into a powerful tool for intentional living.

Each session offers a chance to reflect and recalibrate. Some days are harder than others, but those moments become valuable teachers. They remind us of our strength and resilience, encouraging us to embrace vulnerability. Allowing ourselves to feel every emotion paves the way for healing and growth.

The path ahead is bright, filled with possibilities. With dedication and support, we can continue to thrive. Embracing Wall Pilates opens doors to a deeper understanding of ourselves and our place in the world. The journey unfolds, inviting us to delve into the transformative power of mindful movement, enriching our lives every step of the way.

The Mind-Body Connection

The first element to consider is the principle of the mind-body connection. This connection is fundamental in Pilates, where every movement is performed with full awareness. By nurturing this connection, individuals can reap numerous health benefits. It allows practitioners to become more attuned to their bodies, identifying areas of tension or imbalance that require attention. Enhanced body awareness also promotes better posture and alignment, which are crucial for preventing injuries and alleviating chronic pain. For seniors, this means reducing the risk of falls and maintaining independence, while beginners benefit from building a solid foundation for future exercise endeavors.

Understanding the significance of this connection, therefore, is essential. Studies have shown that practices focusing on the mind-body link, like Pilates, can reduce stress and anxiety levels significantly. By centering one's attention on the present moment and the body's sensations, mindfulness in Wall Pilates creates a meditative state that calms the mind and eases emotional burdens (12 Scientifically Proven Benefits of Pilates for Your Peace of Mind, 2013).

Meditative Focus During Practice

Moving beyond understanding, it's vital to adopt a meditative focus during your Wall Pilates practice. Cultivating this mindset involves integrating brief meditation sessions into your routines. Start your session by closing your eyes and taking a few deep breaths to center yourself. Focus solely on your breathing and let go of any distractions. As you go through your exercises, maintain this focus by continuously bringing your attention back to your breath and the precise movements of your body.

Incorporating short meditation breaks can also be effective. After completing a set of exercises, take a moment to sit quietly and observe any changes in your body. Notice which muscles feel more relaxed and which areas still hold tension. This practice not only enhances the physical benefits of Pilates but also fosters a deeper sense of inner peace and clarity.

Integrating Mindfulness into Routines

To maintain mindfulness throughout your routines, consider establishing specific tactics and reminders. One effective method is setting a clear intention at the beginning of each session. This could be as simple as resolving to stay present or reminding oneself of the goal to connect more deeply with one's body. Visual cues such as placing a note with your intention where you can see it during your practice can serve as constant reminders.

Another tactic involves varying common exercises to keep the mind engaged. For instance, modifying wall squats by incorporating arm raises or adding new elements to familiar moves can prevent the practice from becoming monotonous. These variations challenge both the mind and body, ensuring that each session remains a fresh and stimulating experience.

Positive Affirmations for Connection

Positive affirmations play a crucial role in enhancing the connection between the body and mind during Wall Pilates. Using positive statements can boost self-confidence and create a powerful emotional impact. For example, repeating affirmations like "I am strong and capable" or "I am mindful and present" can reinforce a positive self-image and cultivate a sense of accomplishment. These affirmations can be spoken silently or aloud, depending on what feels most empowering for you.

The benefits of positive affirmations extend beyond the physical practice. They help in framing a constructive mindset that carries over into other aspects of life. Practitioners may notice improved resilience in handling stress and greater ease in navigating daily challenges. For seniors, this might mean feeling more empowered in maintaining their physical health, while beginners may find increased motivation to stick with their fitness journey.

Wall Pilates fosters emotional release and introspection. The slow, controlled movements allow practitioners to tune into their bodies and identify the emotions stored within. You might notice feelings of joy, frustration, or even sadness emerging during your practice. Acknowledging these emotions without judgment is an essential part of the mindfulness journey. It encourages acceptance and self-compassion, which are integral components of holistic well-being.

In addition to structured sessions, incorporating mindfulness into daily routines can sustain its benefits. Simple practices, like mindful walking where you focus on each step and the movement of your legs, can extend the principles of Wall Pilates into everyday life. Similarly, practicing mindful eating by savoring each bite and paying attention to the flavors and textures of food can heighten awareness and appreciation of the present moment.

Overall, Wall Pilates offers a comprehensive approach to fitness that nurtures both the body and mind. By understanding the mind-body connection, adopting a meditative focus, integrating mindfulness into routines, and utilizing positive affirmations, practitioners can achieve a higher level of consciousness in their practice. This holistic approach not only enhances physical health but also fosters mental and emotional well-being, creating a balanced and fulfilling lifestyle.

Concluding Reflections

In this chapter, we have delved into the integration of mindfulness with Wall Pilates, highlighting how mindful breathing techniques can significantly enhance your physical workouts. We explored diaphragmatic breathing and its benefits for both mental clarity and muscle oxygenation. We also looked at the importance of coordinating your breath with movements to maximize effectiveness and reduce injury risks. Additionally, visualization techniques were discussed as a way to keep your mind engaged and foster a positive outlook during exercises.

By incorporating these mindful practices into your Wall Pilates routine, you can transform your workouts into holistic experiences that benefit both body and mind. Practicing consistent, breath-focused routines not only improves physical performance but also develops lasting habits of mindfulness. This approach helps ensure that each exercise session becomes a meaningful and enriching part of your fitness journey, promoting overall well-being and enhancing the quality of your daily life.

Having explored the principles of mindfulness and breathing techniques, we now turn our focus to a crucial aspect of fitness: Wall Pilates routines *specifically* designed for senior fitness. This chapter acknowledges the unique challenges faced by seniors and provides practical modifications to common exercises, ensuring that everyone can participate safely and effectively. By addressing health concerns such as arthritis, balance issues, osteoporosis, and chronic pain, we offer tailored adaptations that not only enhance joint health and functional strength but also promote overall mobility. Through detailed guidance, our goal is to empower seniors to embrace an active lifestyle while minimizing the risk of injury, ultimately enhancing their quality of life.

Chapter 6
Adaptive Workouts for Seniors

Adaptive workouts for seniors involve exercises that cater to their unique needs, ensuring safety and accessibility. By focusing on modifications and low-impact routines, these workouts aim to enhance functional strength, mobility, and overall wellness. Seniors often face challenges due to health conditions like arthritis, balance issues, osteoporosis, and chronic pain, which can limit their ability to engage in traditional fitness regimes. Thus, adapting exercise routines to account for these conditions is crucial for promoting an inclusive fitness environment.

To ensure effectiveness, seniors must understand their limits and listen to their bodies. This means recognizing when a movement feels uncomfortable or causes pain. Instructors who specialize in senior fitness often emphasize the importance of communication during workouts. They encourage participants to share their feelings about certain exercises. When seniors express discomfort, instructors can offer modifications that still allow participants to engage their muscles without risking injury.

Not a senior and skipping this chapter? Make sure to read section 4, "Creating a Sustainable Workout Routine."

Modifications for Common Senior-Specific Conditions

Adapting exercises to meet the unique needs of seniors is crucial for promoting safety, inclusivity, and overall well-being. With age, various health conditions such as arthritis, balance issues, osteoporosis, and chronic pain can affect one's ability to perform physical activities. This section provides practical modifications to Wall Pilates routines that address these common conditions, ensuring that senior fitness remains accessible and effective.

Arthritis-Friendly Adaptations

Arthritis is a prevalent condition among seniors, characterized by joint pain and stiffness. Modifying exercises to accommodate arthritis can help maintain range of motion and alleviate discomfort. Gentle movements and lower-impact variations are essential in these adaptations.

When performing wall-supported squats, reduce the depth to decrease strain on the knees. Instead of bending deeply, seniors can engage in shallow squats while keeping their back against the wall for support. Additionally, incorporating gentle arm circles or shoulder rolls during warm-ups can prepare the joints for movement. These adaptations not only ease joint pain but also encourage participation by making exercises less daunting.

For those with severe arthritis in the hands or wrists, modifying wall push-ups is beneficial. By positioning the hands slightly higher on the wall or using a flat palm instead of fists, pressure on the joints is minimized. Seniors can also use foam blocks to provide cushioning and support. This approach ensures that even individuals with significant joint pain can still engage in upper body strengthening exercises effectively.

Balance Issues Adjustments

Maintaining balance becomes increasingly challenging with age. To address this, specific adaptations can be made to Wall Pilates exercises, providing stability and reducing fall risks. Seated exercises are particularly useful for those with pronounced balance concerns.

Chair-assisted leg lifts are an excellent modification for improving lower body strength while minimizing fall risk. Sitting tall in a chair, seniors can lift one leg at a time, engaging their core muscles to maintain stability. This exercise can be performed slowly to ensure control and balance. Using wall support for standing exercises, such as side leg raises, also offers added stability and confidence. By resting one hand on the wall, seniors can feel secure while working on their leg muscles and enhancing their overall balance.

Incorporating balance-promoting exercises, such as heel-to-toe walking along a wall, allows seniors to practice movement patterns that improve stability. This simple exercise involves placing one foot directly in front of the other, with the wall available for support if needed. Encouraging cautious and controlled movements helps seniors enhance their balance safely without feeling overwhelmed.

Osteoporosis Considerations

Osteoporosis weakens bones, increasing the risk of fractures. Safe exercise practices for seniors with osteoporosis focus on posture, avoiding high-impact movements, and engaging major muscle groups without causing harm.

Weight-bearing exercises, like wall-assisted marches, are effective for maintaining bone density and muscle strength. Standing with their back against the wall, seniors can lift one knee towards their chest while keeping the other foot firmly planted. This controlled movement strengthens the lower body while promoting good posture. Emphasizing proper alignment during these exercises is essential, as slouching or poor form can exacerbate spine issues.

Resistance training using elastic bands is another suitable option. Seniors can attach an elastic band to a sturdy object at shoulder height and perform row-like movements, pulling the band towards their torso. This exercise engages the back muscles and enhances upper body strength without placing excessive stress on the spine.

To further protect the spine, it is vital to avoid forward-flexing exercises like traditional sit-ups. Instead, opt for exercises that maintain a neutral spine position. Gentle back extensions, performed while lying face down and lifting the upper body slightly off the ground, can strengthen the back muscles safely.

Chronic Pain Management

Chronic pain is a persistent issue for many seniors, often limiting their ability to stay active. However, tailored adjustments to Wall Pilates exercises can help manage pain without exacerbating it, contributing to improved wellness and quality of life.

Gentle stretching routines are invaluable for those dealing with chronic pain. Incorporating slow, mindful stretches into the warm-up phase prepares the body for movement. For instance, a wall-supported calf stretch, where seniors place their hands on the wall and step one foot back, can relieve tension in the legs and promote flexibility.

Exercise intensity should be adjusted based on pain levels. On days when pain is more intense, choosing low-impact exercises like seated marches or gentle leg slides against the wall can keep seniors engaged without aggravating their condition. These exercises promote circulation and mobility without putting undue stress on the body.

Encouragement and motivation play pivotal roles in managing chronic pain through exercise. Sharing success stories of individuals who have improved their well-being despite pain can inspire others to stay committed to their fitness journey. Highlighting gradual progress and celebrating small achievements fosters a positive mindset and reinforces the idea that regular, gentle exercise can bring long-term benefits.

Low-Impact Exercises for Joint Health

Introducing low-impact exercises specifically designed to promote joint health is crucial for seniors looking to maintain their mobility and overall well-being. Wall Pilates provides an excellent means to achieve these goals by incorporating modifications that are both gentle on the joints and highly effective in enhancing functional strength. This section will explore a series of accessible exercises, ensuring that each movement is both beneficial and safe for seniors.

Healthy joints allow seniors to move freely and perform everyday tasks without pain. When joint health declines, even simple movements like walking or getting up from a chair can become challenging. This can limit independence and lead to a more sedentary lifestyle. Inactivity can cause muscles to weaken, leading to an increased risk of falls and injuries. Keeping joints healthy helps to ensure that seniors can stay active and engage in social activities, which is key to emotional well-being.

Wall-Assisted Squats

One of the most effective exercises for reinforcing leg strength without placing undue stress on the joints is the wall-assisted squat. This exercise utilizes the support of a wall to ensure proper form and reduce the risk of injury. To perform a wall-assisted squat, stand with your back against the wall and feet shoulder-width apart. Slowly slide down the wall until your knees are bent at a 90-degree angle or as close as comfortable. Hold this position for a few seconds before slowly sliding back up to the starting position.

Wall-assisted squats are particularly beneficial because they allow individuals to strengthen their quadriceps, hamstrings, and glutes while minimizing the impact on the knees and hips. This makes them an ideal choice for seniors who may experience joint pain or stiffness. Additionally, the support provided by the wall helps ensure that the squatting motion is performed correctly, further reducing the likelihood of strain or injury.

Seated Leg Lifts

For those who deal with more pronounced joint pain, seated leg lifts offer an alternative that focuses on enhancing flexibility and promoting circulation. Seated leg lifts can be easily performed using a chair, making them accessible for individuals with varying levels of mobility. To perform this exercise, sit comfortably on a chair with your back straight and feet flat on the floor. Extend one leg forward, keeping it straight but not locked, and hold this position for a few seconds before lowering the leg back to the starting position. Repeat this process with the other leg.

Seated leg lifts provide cumulative benefits for overall mobility and circulation by targeting the lower body muscles without adding stress to the joints. Regular practice of this exercise can lead to improved range of motion in the legs, which is essential for daily activities such as walking and climbing stairs. Over time, the enhanced flexibility gained through seated leg lifts can contribute to greater ease of movement and reduced discomfort during physical activity.

Gentle Wall Presses

Focusing on upper body strength while avoiding strain on the joints can be achieved through gentle wall presses. These exercises are perfect for improving shoulder stability and strength gradually, making them an excellent addition to any senior fitness routine. To perform a gentle wall press, stand facing a wall at arm's length and place your hands flat against the wall at shoulder height. Slowly bend your elbows, bringing your chest closer to the wall, then push back to the starting position.

Gentle wall presses engage the muscles of the shoulders, chest, and arms without subjecting the joints to excessive pressure. This exercise is particularly useful for individuals who may have limited upper body strength and need a low-impact method to build endurance over time. By incorporating variations, such as changing the hand positions or adjusting the distance from the wall, the routine can remain engaging and progressively challenging.

Foot Slide

Engaging the lower body muscles through careful glide exercises, such as the foot slide, can significantly promote joint health while maintaining low exertion levels. The foot slide is an effective way to incorporate gentle movements that are easy to integrate into daily routines. To perform this exercise, stand with one foot slightly in front of the other and place a small towel or slider under the front foot. Slowly slide the foot forward and backward while maintaining balance and control.

The foot slide targets the muscles of the legs, particularly the calves and thighs, and helps improve coordination and balance. This exercise is beneficial because it allows for muscle engagement without adding significant strain to the joints. Regular practice of foot slides can enhance lower body strength and contribute to better stability, which is crucial for preventing falls and maintaining independence.

Guidelines for Safe Exercise Practices

When introducing any new exercise routine, especially for seniors, it's essential to consider specific guidelines to ensure safety and effectiveness. Individuals with osteoporosis should consult with healthcare professionals to tailor exercises that avoid excessive strain on bones while still providing the benefits of strength training (Read, 2024). It's important to focus on maintaining proper posture during exercises to prevent spine injuries and engage major muscle groups safely.

For those dealing with chronic pain, adjustments might be necessary to accommodate individual circumstances. Gentle movements that do not exacerbate pain can help improve overall wellness. It's crucial to listen to one's body and modify the intensity of exercises accordingly. Success stories from others who manage chronic pain through consistent movement can serve as motivation and empowerment for seniors embarking on similar journeys.

Building Functional Strength and Mobility

Building functional strength and improving mobility is essential for seniors, and Wall Pilates exercises provide a tailored approach to meeting these goals. Staying strong allows seniors to carry out daily activities with greater ease. Simple tasks like lifting groceries or standing up from a chair become less daunting when strength is enhanced. Increased strength also reduces the risk of falls, one of the leading causes of serious injury among older adults. When seniors feel secure in their movements, they are more likely to engage in social activities, leading to improved mental well-being.

Improving mobility is just as crucial. As flexibility and range of motion increase, seniors can move more freely. This can lead to a greater sense of independence. For instance, bending to tie a shoe or reaching for items on a high shelf becomes achievable. Enhanced mobility allows seniors to participate in activities they enjoy, whether it's gardening, walking in the park, or playing with grandchildren. When they can move without pain or stiffness, their overall quality of life improves dramatically.

Wall Pilates focuses on building strength and mobility in a safe and supportive way. This method often emphasizes core strength, balance, and controlled movements, which are essential for everyday functions. The wall provides stability, making exercises more accessible and less intimidating. Each pose and movement can be adjusted to fit individual needs, allowing seniors to progress at their own pace. This personalized approach ensures that they can enjoy the benefits without the fear of overexerting themselves.

This section explores core stability exercises, wall push-ups for upper body strength, hip openers and stretching, and functional reach exercises. Each of these components plays a vital role in maintaining overall wellness and enhancing daily life activities.

Core Stability Exercises

Core stability is foundational to maintaining overall body function and balance, especially for seniors. Simple exercises targeting the core, such as wall-assisted pelvic tilts and seated leg lifts, can significantly enhance core engagement. Pelvic tilts involve standing with your back against the wall, tilting your pelvis forward and then back, while focusing on tightening the abdominal muscles. This exercise helps in strengthening the lower back and abdominal muscles, which are crucial for stability and posture.

Seated leg lifts, performed while sitting in a chair close to the wall, emphasize lower abdominal strength. By lifting one leg at a time while keeping the core engaged, individuals can improve their ability to rise from chairs or beds more easily. The key is consistency and proper form, ensuring that each movement is controlled and deliberate to maximize benefits without causing strain.

Wall Push-Ups for Upper Body Strength

Upper body strength can be safely developed through modified wall push-ups. Unlike traditional push-ups, wall push-ups use the support of a wall, making them an excellent option for seniors who may find floor exercises challenging. To perform a wall push-up, stand facing the wall with arms extended and hands placed at shoulder height. Slowly bend your elbows to bring your chest closer to the wall, then push back to the starting position.

This exercise not only strengthens the arms and shoulders but also engages the chest and upper back —muscle groups used in everyday activities like lifting groceries or pushing doors open. Consistent practice can lead to improved upper body strength, enhancing the ability to perform daily tasks independently and confidently.

Hip Openers and Stretching

Gentle hip-opening exercises are crucial for enhancing mobility and preventing stiffness, especially in seniors. Exercises such as wall-supported hip flexor stretches can be particularly beneficial. Stand next to the wall for balance, place one foot forward, and gently push your hips down and forward to stretch the hip flexors. Hold the stretch for a few seconds before switching legs.

Another effective exercise is the seated figure-four stretch, where you sit in a chair, cross one ankle over the opposite knee, and gently press down on the crossed knee. This helps in opening up the hip joint and relieving tension. Incorporating these stretches into regular routines can improve flexibility, reduce the risk of injuries, and ease movements during daily activities.

Functional Reach Exercises

Functional reach exercises mimic daily tasks, providing practical benefits by directly translating exercise movements into real-life improvements. One such exercise involves standing near the wall, reaching one arm up and out as if trying to grab an object from a high shelf. This not only enhances shoulder and arm flexibility but also boosts confidence in performing similar tasks at home.

Another example is the wall-supported side reach. Stand sideways to the wall with one hand on it for support, then extend your other arm overhead and lean towards the wall. This exercise stretches the side of the body and improves reach capability, helping with tasks like reaching into cupboards or hanging clothes. Functional reach exercises foster independence and assure seniors of their physical capabilities, boosting overall well-being.

Creating a Sustainable Workout Routine

Creating a sustainable workout routine is essential for achieving long-term fitness goals and maintaining overall health. For both seniors seeking to enhance their mobility and younger individuals aiming to build strength, establishing a consistent Wall Pilates practice can provide numerous benefits. The challenge often lies in staying motivated and ensuring the routine remains engaging and effective over time. A well-structured approach that includes setting achievable targets, incorporating variety, and fostering accountability can greatly enhance the likelihood of success.

Sticking to a routine helps to build consistency. When you have a set schedule, it becomes easier to stick with your plan. You know what to expect and when to do it. This regularity helps form a habit, making it less daunting to get started each day. The body also responds better to consistent training. Muscles adapt to the stress you place on them, leading to improved strength and endurance over time. Without a routine, it's easy to skip workouts or lose motivation.

A routine also allows for better tracking of progress. You can measure improvements in strength, endurance, or flexibility over time. Tracking your workouts helps to see what works best for you and where you need to adjust. Recording achievements, even small ones, can boost morale. It feels rewarding to hit milestones, such as lifting heavier weights or running longer distances. Seeing tangible results can motivate you to continue.

A structured routine can also help prevent injuries. When you follow a plan, you have a balance of training and rest days that minimizes the risk of overworking any one part of the body. It allows muscle groups to recover. Recovery is just as important as the workouts themselves. Without proper recovery, one can easily become fatigued or strained, which can lead to setbacks.

Setting Achievable Goals

Setting realistic fitness targets is a crucial step in creating and maintaining a sustainable Wall Pilates routine. Establishing achievable goals can help keep you motivated and on track, reducing the risk of feeling overwhelmed or discouraged. Understanding how to set these targets effectively allows for steady progress, ensuring that you can continue to enjoy the benefits of your workout routine.

To begin, it's essential to empower yourself by defining clear and specific fitness aspirations. When setting goals, consider what you genuinely want to achieve through your Wall Pilates practice. Are you looking to improve your balance, enhance your flexibility, or build functional strength? Identifying your primary objectives will provide direction and purpose to your workouts. For seniors aged 60 and above, this might mean focusing on exercises that enhance mobility and protect joint health. For younger beginners, it might mean building core strength and endurance.

Once you have identified your fitness aspirations, it's critical to recognize the importance of small steps for steady progress. Breaking down large goals into smaller, manageable tasks can make them feel less daunting and more attainable. For instance, instead of aiming to perform a complex Wall Pilates move perfectly right away, start with mastering its basic components. This approach ensures that each workout contributes to your overall progress, fostering a sense of achievement and momentum.

Celebrating milestones along your fitness journey is another vital aspect of maintaining motivation. Recognizing and acknowledging improvements, no matter how small, can significantly boost your enthusiasm and commitment. Whether it's being able to hold a plank position for a few seconds longer, achieving better posture, or simply feeling more energized after your workouts, these victories matter. Consider keeping a journal to track your accomplishments and reflect on your progress regularly. Sharing these achievements with friends or loved ones can also provide additional encouragement and support.

Regularly reviewing and adjusting your goals based on your progress is another important strategy. Periodic assessments allow you to evaluate what's working well and identify areas where you might need to make changes. Setting aside time every few weeks to revisit your fitness targets ensures that they remain relevant and aligned with your current abilities and aspirations. This practice helps prevent stagnation and keeps you engaged with your Wall Pilates routine.

Establishing realistic fitness targets involves a thoughtful process. Begin by defining your fitness aspirations and breaking them down into smaller, manageable steps. Celebrate milestones to maintain motivation and be adaptable as your fitness levels evolve. Regularly review and adjust your goals to ensure they remain relevant and achievable. By following these strategies, you will be better equipped to create a sustainable Wall Pilates routine that promotes continuous progress and long-term success.

Incorporating Variety

Creating a sustainable Wall Pilates routine is more than just following a set of exercises; it requires creativity, personal assessment, and social support to maintain engagement and consistency. For seniors aiming to enhance functional strength, flexibility, and balance, as well as for beginner fitness enthusiasts looking to establish a consistent routine, these elements are crucial.

First, let's consider the role of creativity in combining different Wall Pilates movements. To avoid monotony, it's essential to mix various exercises. By doing so, you not only keep your mind engaged but also target different muscle groups, leading to a more balanced workout. For example, you could start with a gentle wall roll-down to warm up, followed by wall squats for leg strength, and finish with a wall plank for core stability. The variation ensures that you are not doing the same movements repeatedly, which can become tedious and reduce motivation. Experimenting with new combinations can make the practice feel fresh and exciting.

To encourage creativity, try setting aside time each week to research new Wall Pilates exercises or ask an instructor for recommendations. Create a list of various movements and mix them up to design a routine that changes every few sessions.

Another important aspect is assessing which exercises work best for you. This personal evaluation enhances both enjoyment and accountability. Everyone's body reacts differently to specific exercises, and what works wonders for one person might be less effective or even uncomfortable for another. Pay attention to how your body feels during and after each exercise. Do certain movements leave you feeling invigorated, while others cause discomfort? Make a note of these reactions and adjust your routine accordingly. This tailored approach ensures that you look forward to your workouts and remain committed.

Building Accountability

Let's delve into the power of shared experiences and community engagement. These factors can significantly bolster your commitment to a fitness routine. Being part of a community, whether local or online, provides a sense of belonging and accountability. Sharing your progress and challenges with others facing similar journeys can be incredibly motivating. You might discover that discussing a particularly tough move becomes easier when you realize others have struggled with it too. This shared experience fosters camaraderie and perseverance.

Community engagement can take many forms. Local classes offer immediate interaction and support. They allow you to receive instant feedback from instructors and encouragement from fellow participants. On the other hand, online groups provide flexibility and access to a global community. You can join forums, attend virtual classes, or participate in social media challenges. These platforms allow you to share achievements, seek advice, and stay connected regardless of geographical constraints.

Don't underestimate the value of simply sharing your goals with friends or family. Letting those close to you know about your fitness ambitions can create a supportive environment. Friends or family members can offer encouragement and recognize your efforts, making it challenging to skip workouts. You may even inspire them to join you, fostering a shared commitment to health and fitness.

Scheduling Workouts

To further explore ways to incorporate Wall Pilates into daily life, consider using reminders or fitness apps. Technology can be a valuable ally in maintaining consistency. Set daily or weekly reminders on your phone or calendar to prompt you to exercise. There are numerous apps designed specifically for tracking workouts, offering a range of features such as exercise demonstrations, progress logs, and motivational messages. These tools help keep you accountable and provide structure, making it easier to integrate Wall Pilates into your busy schedule.

Try incorporating a fitness app to track your Wall Pilates sessions. Utilize features that allow you to set goals, monitor progress, and receive reminders. This external prompt can be particularly useful in establishing and maintaining a consistent routine.

It's important to remember that every little effort contributes to progress over time. Even if you can't commit to a full workout session every day, short bursts of activity can still make a difference. Incorporate Wall Pilates moves into your daily routine – maybe a few minutes while waiting for the kettle to boil or during TV commercial breaks. These small actions accumulate and lead to improved strength and flexibility.

Find ways to integrate Wall Pilates into your everyday tasks. Perform quick exercises while waiting for dinner to cook or during short breaks throughout your day. Consistent, manageable efforts can lead to significant long-term benefits.

Incorporating these Wall Pilates exercises into daily routines offers significant benefits for seniors, emphasizing the importance of functional strength and mobility. Regular practice of core stability exercises ensures a strong foundation, making every move safer and more efficient. Wall push-ups offer a gentle yet effective way to build upper body strength, crucial for various daily activities. Hip openers and stretches ward off stiffness and enhance flexibility, allowing for easier, pain-free movements. Lastly, functional reach exercises empower seniors to perform day-to-day tasks with confidence and ease.

For those seeking to maintain or improve their fitness levels, Wall Pilates presents an accessible, low-impact option. Its modifications cater to diverse physical abilities, making it suitable for both active seniors and beginner fitness enthusiasts. The added support of the wall provides stability, reducing the risk of falls and injuries, which is especially important for older adults.

Staying active through Wall Pilates can help manage and even prevent chronic conditions. Regular exercise has been shown to have numerous health benefits, including better management of diabetes, heart problems, and high blood pressure. For seniors, being physically active can lead to improved mental health, reduced risk of dementia, and easier recovery from illness or injury.

Working these exercises into a consistent routine can lead to gradual but noticeable improvements in strength, flexibility, and balance. This commitment to regular activity promotes longevity and enhances the quality of life. The aim is not just to stay fit but to live independently and confidently, enjoying the daily activities that contribute to a fulfilling life.

Harnessing What You've Learned

Throughout this chapter, we have explored various modifications to Wall Pilates exercises designed to accommodate common senior-specific conditions such as arthritis, balance issues, osteoporosis, and chronic pain. By tailoring these routines with low-impact adaptations, seniors can safely enhance their functional strength, mobility, and overall wellness. Emphasizing proper posture, controlled movements, and inclusive practices ensures that individuals of all abilities can participate in these beneficial activities while minimizing the risk of injury or discomfort.

These thoughtful modifications not only make fitness more accessible but also promote a sense of confidence and independence among seniors. Incorporating seated exercises, gentle stretching, and mindful adjustments based on individual pain levels allows for a customized approach that caters to diverse needs. The ultimate goal is to foster a sustainable fitness routine that supports healthy aging, improves daily functioning, and enhances the quality of life for seniors and beginner fitness enthusiasts alike.

Next, we'll shift the focus to the development of Wall Pilates programs designed for a broader audience, encompassing entry-level to intermediate participants. Here, we will explore essential techniques that not only introduce foundational movements but also guide you in incrementally increasing the intensity of your workouts. As you learn to track your progress and set tangible milestones, you'll find renewed motivation to continue your fitness journey. The ultimate goal is to equip you with the necessary tools to create a safe and effective workout plan that adapts and evolves with your growing abilities, fostering a lifelong commitment to health and wellness.

Chapter 7
Progressive Workouts for Beginners

Designing workouts that cater to beginners requires a thoughtful approach that emphasizes gradual progression and motivation. Progressive workouts introduce fitness enthusiasts to the basics, ensuring that they build a solid foundation before advancing to more complex routines. This strategy not only helps in preventing injuries but also promotes steady improvements in strength, flexibility, and confidence.

Creating progressive workouts is essential for beginners because it helps one develop a strong connection to exercise. When newcomers feel successful at their level, they are more likely to stick with their routines. Small, achievable goals help increase their motivation and establish a rhythm that keeps them engaged. For instance, instead of jumping into intense workouts right away, a beginner can start by walking or doing simple bodyweight exercises. This creates a positive experience rather than an overwhelming one.

Progressive workouts also emphasize the importance of proper technique and form. Beginners often benefit from guidance to ensure they are executing movements correctly. Using resources like personal trainers, instructional videos, or even group classes assists one in avoiding common mistakes. Learning the right techniques early on builds confidence, making it easier for beginners to progress to more challenging exercises. Safety should always be a priority, and knowing how to perform exercises correctly protects one from injuries.

Finally, being patient with oneself is key. Progress takes time, and celebrating small victories can help keep one's spirits up. Whether it's increasing the weight one can lift or completing an additional five minutes of cardio, recognizing these achievements reinforces one's hard work. Reminding beginners that fitness is a lifelong journey can help one embrace the process and remain dedicated to one's goals.

Progressive workouts are essential tools for beginners, guiding one on one's fitness journey. They offer a supportive and gradual approach that promotes health and well-being. When beginners feel empowered, motivated, and informed, they are more likely to remain committed and share their love for fitness with others. The impact of this positive experience can resonate far beyond their initial workouts, ultimately transforming their lives for the better.

Gradual Progression Strategies

Gradual progression is a cornerstone of safe and effective Wall Pilates practice, particularly for beginners. It ensures that participants build their strength, flexibility, and confidence in a structured manner without overloading their bodies. For seniors aged 60 and above, as well as beginner fitness enthusiasts aged 20 to 50, mastering the basics before moving on to more advanced exercises is critical.

One of the first concepts to understand is the importance of mastering foundational movements before attempting advanced modifications. Foundational movements such as wall planks, wall squats, and lateral wall slides serve as the building blocks of more complex routines. These exercises not only help improve balance and stability but also reinforce proper form and technique. By focusing on these basic movements initially, practitioners can avoid common injuries associated with improper alignment and muscle strain.

- **Wall planks** are straightforward yet effective. Start by finding a clear wall and standing a few feet away from it. Place your hands on the wall at shoulder height, keeping your arms straight. Walk your feet back until your body forms a straight line from head to heels. Engage your core and hold this position. The goal is to maintain a straight and strong posture for as long as you can. Ensure your shoulders are directly above your wrists and breathe steadily. Aim to hold the plank for at least 10-20 seconds.

- **Wall squats** require you to find a sturdy wall. Stand with your back against it and feet shoulder-width apart, about two feet away from the wall. Slowly slide down the wall until your thighs are parallel to the ground, similar to sitting in an invisible chair. Keep your back pressed against the wall and your knees aligned over your ankles. Hold this position, engaging your thighs and glutes. To start, hold for 15 to 30 seconds, then push back up to a standing position. Gradually increase the hold time as you gain strength.

- **Lateral wall slides** focus on upper body mobility. Stand with your back against the wall, feet shoulder-width apart. Your arms should be raised to shoulder height, bent at the elbows, and pressed flat against the wall. Slowly slide your arms up over your head, keeping them in contact with the wall. Once your arms are extended, slide them back down to the starting position. This movement helps strengthen the shoulders while improving flexibility. Perform this for 10 to 15 repetitions, focusing on smooth and controlled movements.

For seniors, this approach offers a gentle introduction to exercise, while younger beginners benefit from developing a robust foundation. For instance, wall squats can be started at a shallow depth, gradually increasing as strength and confidence build. This methodical approach allows individuals to experience the benefits of each exercise fully before transitioning to more challenging variations.

Incremental changes in intensity also play a significant role in building confidence and skill. When starting with Wall Pilates, it's important to begin with minimal resistance and few repetitions. As proficiency increases, adding elements such as holding poses longer or increasing the repetitions helps to gradually intensify the workout. This measured progression ensures that the body adapts without feeling overwhelmed.

To illustrate, consider wall planks, which are excellent for core strengthening. Beginners might start by holding a plank for just ten seconds, then slowly increase the duration as they become more comfortable. This gradual increase not only promotes physical endurance but also enhances mental resilience, encouraging participants to push their boundaries safely.

Documenting progress serves as both a motivational tool and a practical guide for improvement. Keeping a record of workouts, including the types of exercises performed, duration, intensity, and personal reflections, provides tangible evidence of advancement. For many, seeing measurable progress boosts motivation and reinforces commitment to regular practice. A journal or a fitness app can be instrumental in tracking improvements and identifying areas needing attention.

For instance, seniors might note improvements in daily activities such as easier bending to tie shoes or reduced stiffness upon waking. Younger beginners may document increased stamina during workouts or better posture throughout the day. This practice not only keeps participants engaged but also helps tailor subsequent sessions to address specific needs or achieve targeted goals.

With these principles in mind, setting up a structured Wall Pilates program becomes more manageable. An initial routine might include five to ten minutes of basic exercises, such as wall angels for shoulder mobility, followed by wall squats and lateral wall slides. Over time, as comfort and ability levels rise, additional exercises like single-leg wall squats or advanced wall planks can be integrated. The objective is to ensure that each session builds on the last, creating a seamless transition from basic to more advanced practices.

- To perform **wall angels** , stand with your back against a wall. Ensure your feet are about six inches away from the wall, and your lower back, shoulders, and head are touching it. Raise your arms to form a "Y" shape, and slide them up and down the wall, keeping your elbows and wrists in contact with the surface. This movement opens up the chest and shoulders, enhancing mobility.

- As proficiency grows, **single-leg wall squats** become a great addition. Begin in the wall squat position, then lift one leg off the ground while still keeping your back against the wall. Lower into a squat on the standing leg while ensuring it remains stable. This move enhances balance and strengthens each leg independently.

- **Advanced wall planks** require getting into a plank position with your feet against the wall. Your hands should be on the ground, aligning with your shoulders. Engage your core and hold the position, ensuring your body forms a straight line from head to heels. Start with shorter holds and gradually increase as strength improves. This exercise targets the core and shoulders, developing overall stability.

Integrate these exercises in a way that allows your body to adapt and progress at a comfortable pace. Start with two sets of ten repetitions for each exercise, and as you get stronger, aim to increase the number of sets or incorporate weights. Pay attention to your form and breathing during each movement, which is critical for achieving the best results.

Listening to one's body is essential during this journey. While the roadmap encourages steady progression, everyone's pace will vary. It's vital to recognize and respect individual limits to prevent burnout or injury. Fatigue or discomfort signals that it may be time to rest or modify an exercise.

This approach aligns well with the overall goal of enhancing functional strength, flexibility, and balance without causing undue stress or injury. By pacing themselves, seniors and beginners alike can find enjoyment and satisfaction in their Pilates practice, fostering a lifelong commitment to health and wellness.

Combining Cardio with Wall Pilates

Integrating cardio elements into Wall Pilates can significantly enhance overall fitness, particularly for those beginning their journey or seeking a low-impact routine to maintain functional strength and flexibility. Cardio exercises are vital as they effectively increase heart rate and improve circulation, working hand-in-hand with the core-strengthening benefits of Wall Pilates.

Firstly, cardio exercises elevate the heart rate and boost circulation, which is important for cardiovascular health. Activities like wall-supported kicks and gentle marching in place while leaning on a wall serve as effective entry points for beginners. These movements not only raise the heart rate but also provide dynamic engagement, fostering better blood flow throughout the body. This enhanced circulation ensures that muscles receive more oxygen and nutrients, promoting quicker recovery and reducing muscle fatigue.

- Perform **wall-supported kicks** by standing with your feet hip-width apart. Place your hands on the wall for balance. Lift one leg straight out in front of you, then lower it back down. Repeat this motion for several repetitions before switching to the other leg. Try to keep a steady rhythm. Focus on your posture; ensure your back is straight and your stomach is tight. You can perform this with a small pause between each kick for better control.

- For **gentle marching in place** , start by standing tall and placing your hands on the wall. Begin to lift your knees alternately, as if you are walking in place. Keep your movements slow and controlled to avoid losing balance. Try to raise each knee to about waist level. You can vary the speed to match your comfort level. This also helps activate your core.

Incorporating low-impact cardio options like gentle marching or wall-supported kicks is especially beneficial for those new to exercise or individuals with joint concerns. Low-impact exercises reduce stress on the joints while still providing the cardiovascular benefits necessary for a balanced workout.

Boosting endurance through mindful integration of cardio into Wall Pilates complements the existing focus on flexibility and strength training. Endurance is built gradually by incorporating short bursts of cardio between traditional Wall Pilates exercises. For example, alternating between wall squats and brisk wall marches can create an effective circuit. This approach not only enhances muscular endurance but also keeps the heart rate elevated, ensuring a comprehensive workout that addresses multiple aspects of fitness simultaneously.

Creating simple routines that blend both disciplines encourages variety and enjoyment, making workouts more engaging and less monotonous. A well-crafted routine might start with a set of wall push-ups to engage the upper body, followed by a minute of gentle marching to elevate the heart rate. Next, wall sits can target the lower body muscles, paired with wall-supported kicks to maintain cardiovascular activity. This pattern continues, merging the benefits of strength, flexibility, and cardio, creating a balanced and enjoyable exercise experience.

An example routine could look as follows:

- **Wall Push-ups** : Begin with 10 repetitions, focusing on controlled breathing to engage the chest, shoulders, and triceps.

- **Gentle Marching** : Transition into 1 minute of gentle marching in place, using the wall for support to ensure stability.

- **Wall Sits** : Move to 15 seconds of wall sits, keeping the back flat against the wall and bending the knees at a right angle to strengthen the legs and glutes.

- **Wall-supported Kicks** : Follow up with 10 kicks per leg. Lift and extend one leg slowly to work on hip flexibility and strength.

- **Wall Squats** : Perform 10 wall squats to further engage the lower body, ensuring proper form to protect the knees.

- **Brisk Wall Marches** : Conclude with another minute of brisk wall marches, maintaining a steady pace to keep the heart rate elevated.

The variety in these exercises not only prevents boredom but also ensures that different muscle groups are engaged, providing a holistic workout experience.

Integrating wearable weights or resistance bands can add an extra challenge once the basic exercises become too easy. For instance, wearing light ankle weights during wall-supported kicks increases resistance, further enhancing muscle tone and cardiovascular effort. Resistance bands can be used during wall squats to add tension and improve lower body strength.

Regularly practicing this combined approach helps in building a strong foundation of cardiovascular fitness, muscular endurance, and flexibility. Over time, as endurance improves, the duration and intensity of the cardio intervals can be increased to continue challenging the body and making progress.

Studies show that mixing cardio with strength training leads to superior fitness outcomes compared to either modality alone. This underscores the importance of an integrated exercise approach, particularly for seniors aiming to maintain functional strength and younger individuals developing a consistent fitness routine.

Tracking Progress with Measurable Goals

Setting and tracking measurable fitness goals is essential for anyone beginning a workout regimen, particularly for those new to Wall Pilates. Establishing clear, attainable targets not only provides direction but also fuels motivation as progress is observed. To fully equip readers with practical tools for this purpose, we delve into effective strategies for goal setting and the importance of consistent tracking.

One vital reason for setting goals is the boost in accountability it provides. Sharing fitness goals with a friend or community can create a sense of responsibility. When someone knows that others are aware of their targets, they are more likely to stay committed. Accountability partners can cheer each other on, offer valuable advice, and help keep motivation levels high. It makes the journey less lonely and more engaging, as there is someone to share both struggles and victories with.

Once you have set achievable goals, it's beneficial to break them down into smaller, more manageable steps. This process helps in staying focused and motivated, as these small wins accumulate over time. For example, if your goal is to improve your core strength, you can start by mastering one basic Wall Pilates move before gradually increasing the complexity and number of repetitions. This step-by-step approach not only makes the journey less daunting but also allows for regular moments of success, which can be incredibly motivating.

Goal setting goes hand in hand with self-compassion. As you encounter obstacles or experience setbacks, remind yourself that it's a part of the journey. Instead of viewing difficulties as failures, look at them as opportunities to learn and grow. Adjusting goals in response to these challenges demonstrates resilience and commitment to your overall fitness journey.

Maintaining a positive mindset can significantly impact your ability to achieve your fitness goals. Visualization techniques—envisioning yourself successfully reaching your targets—can play a powerful role. Imagining yourself completing a workout, mastering a new move, or simply feeling healthier can make the goals feel more attainable and drive you forward.

Ultimately, the journey towards achieving fitness goals is deeply personal. Each individual has unique aspirations and challenges, and it's essential to honor that individuality. Customizing your approach and embracing what works best for you will create an enjoyable experience. Whether you're aiming to enhance your strength, improve flexibility, or simply find joy in movement, the most critical aspect is to keep pursuing your goals with enthusiasm and determination.

Understanding the SMART Criteria for Fitness Goals

Setting fitness goals can sometimes feel overwhelming. However, using the SMART criteria can help in creating a clear and effective approach. The SMART criteria consist of five important elements: Specific, Measurable, Achievable, Relevant, and Time-bound. Each element plays a critical role in guiding you through your fitness journey, ensuring that you stay focused and motivated.

Specific Goals

The first step in setting fitness goals is ensuring they are specific. A vague goal such as "getting fit" doesn't give you much direction. Instead, consider what "getting fit" really means to you. For example, you could aim to "improve core strength" or "increase endurance." A clear, specific goal might be "improve core strength by practicing Wall Pilates for 20 minutes daily." This gives you a clear target. Knowing exactly what you want to accomplish makes it easier to create a plan and track your progress.

To set specific goals, start by asking yourself a few questions. What do I want to achieve? Why is this goal important to me? When do I want to achieve it? These questions help clarify what exactly you're aiming for. For instance, improving your core strength can benefit activities like running, swimming, or even day-to-day tasks like lifting groceries.

Measurable Goals

Once you have a specific goal in mind, the next step is to make it measurable. This means defining how you will track your progress. Having measurable goals gives you tangible ways to see how you're improving. For instance, if your specific goal is to hold a plank position for two minutes, you can measure your current time and set mini-goals to improve gradually. You might start by holding a plank for 30 seconds and aim to increase that by 10 seconds each week.

Another approach to measuring progress is keeping a journal or using apps designed for tracking workouts. Write down your results weekly. You can note improvements in holding a plank position or list how many repetitions of an exercise you can now complete. This record helps reinforce that change is happening, building motivation along the way.

Achievable Goals

Setting goals that are achievable is another crucial component of the SMART criteria. It's great to have ambitious targets, but if your goals are too far out of reach, you might feel discouraged. Instead, consider what is realistic based on your current fitness level. If you are new to exercising, looking to jump straight into high-intensity training might not make sense. Instead, set smaller, incremental goals. For instance, if your aim is to run a 5K, start by walking for 10 minutes daily and gradually build up to jogging.

When setting achievable goals, think about what resources you have. Do you have access to a gym? Can you work out at home? Taking small steps is essential in building confidence. Celebrate small victories, like completing a week of workouts. Each little achievement inspires you to keep going and proves that you are making progress.

Relevant Goals

The next element of the SMART criteria is ensuring your goals are relevant. This means that your fitness goals should align with your personal interests and larger life objectives. Ask yourself how this goal fits into your life and if it brings you joy or serves a purpose. For example, if you dream of enhancing your flexibility and functional strength, concentrate on exercises that support these ambitions. Choosing relevant goals ensures you are excited and motivated to work toward them.

Consider different aspects of fitness that are significant for you. If you enjoy outdoor activities like hiking or biking, set goals that improve your performance in those areas. This alignment leads to a more fulfilling workout experience, making you less likely to stray from your routine.

Time-bound Goals

Lastly, making your goals time-bound is essential for creating a sense of urgency. Without a deadline, it is easy to procrastinate or lose focus. Choose a specific timeframe for your goals. For example, you might aim to reach a certain level of proficiency within three months or target an upcoming event, like a charity run. By having a schedule, you can divide your main goal into weekly or monthly milestones.

For example, if your goal is to run a 5K in three months, break it down into a weekly running regimen. You might dedicate the first month to building your base endurance, focusing on regular walking and short jogging sessions. In the following months, increase your distance each week until you are ready to run the 5K. Keeping the timeline in mind will act as a motivating factor, encouraging you to remain consistent and committed.

Setting fitness goals using the SMART criteria helps create a structured path for improvement. By ensuring your goals are Specific, Measurable, Achievable, Relevant, and Time-bound, you establish clarity in your objectives. This structured approach keeps you motivated, allowing you to enjoy your fitness journey more thoroughly. Remember that the journey to fitness is not just about reaching the destination but also about the growth and experiences along the way.

Progress Tracking

Documenting achievements is a very important part of tracking progress in any fitness journey. Keeping a record of what you accomplish helps you see just how far you've come. It also shows you the areas where you might need to improve. There are many ways to document your fitness journey, including using journals, mobile applications, or community platforms. Each method has its own benefits that can make tracking progress easier and more effective.

A fitness journal is a simple yet effective tool for recording your daily exercises. With a journal, you write down everything you do during workouts. For example, you can note the number of repetitions for each exercise or how long you spend on different activities. You might also want to describe any feelings or physical sensations you experience during or after exercising. Sometimes, you might feel tired; other times, you might feel energized. By writing down these details, you're not just keeping a record but also reflecting on your experiences. This can help you understand how your body responds to different workouts, allowing you to adjust your routine as needed.

When you look back at your progress in a journal, it can be very motivating. It's rewarding to see all that you've achieved laid out in front of you. You might find that you can do more repetitions than when you started or that your workouts last longer. This visual evidence can encourage you to keep pushing forward. Knowing that your hard work is paying off can boost your confidence and inspire you to set bigger goals for yourself.

Mobile applications provide a modern twist on the way you can track your fitness progress. Many of these apps come with features designed to make the tracking process smoother. For instance, some apps can automatically log your workouts for you. This means you don't have to remember to enter everything manually. Many also offer reminders to keep you on track with your fitness goals. This is very helpful if you have a busy schedule and tend to forget about your workout plans.

Visualizing your progress over time is another great feature of these apps. They often include graphs or charts that show how your performance improves. For example, you might see a graph that displays your increasing endurance or strength levels. This visual representation makes it easier to see changes that happen over weeks and months. Seeing these figures can provide a clearer picture of your fitness journey and help you stay motivated.

Community platforms are another fantastic way to track your progress. They allow you to connect with others on similar fitness journeys. Engaging with friends or even strangers who share similar goals can add a social element to your fitness routine. When you share your achievements with the community, it allows you to celebrate your successes together. This sense of belonging helps you feel more committed to your goals.

On these platforms, you can also exchange tips and advice with others. If you're struggling with a particular exercise or not sure how to stay motivated, someone else might share what works for them. Having this support network can make a huge difference. You can learn new techniques, discover workout ideas you hadn't thought about, and even find workout partners. Together, you can encourage each other to stay consistent and reach new milestones.

Using a combination of these methods can create a comprehensive approach to tracking your fitness journey. You might find that writing regularly in a journal works well for your day-to-day reflection. At the same time, an app might help you visualize your progress with graphs and reminders. Engaging with a community can add motivation and accountability, making your journey feel less isolated.

As you document your experiences, always remember to celebrate your victories, no matter how small. Whether you managed to run an extra mile or lifted a slightly heavier weight, each achievement deserves recognition. Acknowledging your progress, even in minor ways, can significantly boost your motivation. It can push you to keep reaching for bigger goals and striving for improvement.

Progress tracking is not solely about the numbers. It's also about creating a deeper understanding of your body and how it responds to various types of exercise. By keeping a close eye on your journey, you can identify patterns. Maybe you notice that certain workouts leave you feeling more energized than others. Understanding these patterns can enable you to tailor your fitness routine better to meet your needs.

It's also important to reflect on and adjust your goals as you progress. Your initial goal might have been to run a 5K, but as you make progress, you might find yourself motivated to aim for a 10K or half marathon. Having that ability to adjust your focus keeps things fresh. It can prevent the process from becoming stale, helping you stay engaged and interested in your fitness journey.

Incorporating these various methods into your routine can turn progress tracking into a fulfilling process. With tools like journals, apps, and community support, you can effectively monitor your growth. The act of documenting what you achieve contributes significantly to your fitness success and can keep you motivated through ups and downs. As you progress, remember that every step forward, no matter how big or small, is a part of your unique journey toward fitness and well-being.

Reflective Practice

Reflective practice is a vital part of your fitness journey. It involves taking the time to think about your progress and understand where you are in your fitness goals. Reflection is more than just looking back; it helps you identify areas that may need improvement. This might include adjusting your workout routines or changing your nutritional habits. Regularly checking in with yourself allows you to see what is working well and what areas might not be contributing to your overall fitness journey.

When you engage in reflective practice, you also acknowledge that setbacks are normal. Everyone experiences challenges, whether it's missing a workout or not seeing the expected results. These moments should not discourage you. Instead, they are a natural part of the growth process. For instance, if you find that your weight has plateaued for a while, rather than feeling defeated, consider revisiting your workout plan. Perhaps it's time to add new exercises, increase the intensity, or even take a break and allow your body to recover. By understanding that setbacks can lead to growth, you can maintain a more positive mindset.

As you reflect on your journey, take note of the specific exercises that contribute positively or negatively to your goals. For example, if you notice that a particular workout isn't helping you improve your strength or endurance, it's a sign that you should re-evaluate. Perhaps you are not performing the exercises correctly, or maybe they are simply not suitable for your fitness level. This reflection helps you make informed choices. You can choose to seek guidance from a trainer or even research proper techniques online so you can execute the exercises correctly.

Reflective practice can guide you in setting new goals. Once you have recognized your progress, it's important to set new targets to aim for. This could be anything from increasing your weights, trying a new class, or even signing up for a fun run. Clear goals give you something concrete to work towards, making your journey feel more structured. For instance, if you want to work on your flexibility, you might decide to incorporate yoga into your routine three times a week. Setting specific, measurable goals keeps you accountable and gives your workouts a sense of purpose.

Seeking feedback from others can enhance your reflective practice. Talking to friends, family, or a fitness coach can provide new perspectives on your progress. They might notice things you haven't or suggest modifications that can help you improve. For instance, if you share your experiences with a friend who is also into fitness, they could give you valuable insight into their own journey that might apply to yours. Sometimes, a different viewpoint can open up new avenues for growth and improvement.

Incorporating technology can also support your reflective practice. There are numerous apps that allow you to track your workouts, monitor your progress, and even analyze your performance. By regularly inputting your fitness data, you can look back at trends and patterns in your training. This data-driven approach provides concrete evidence of your progress and can assist in making informed decisions about your fitness plan. It can highlight areas that are improving over time and those that may need additional focus.

Each part of the reflective process contributes to a deeper understanding of your fitness journey. Whether it's understanding your setbacks or celebrating your victories, reflection allows you to stay engaged. It helps you see your journey as a whole rather than just isolated moments. This holistic view can transform how you approach fitness, allowing you to embrace the process and enjoy the ride.

Reflective practice is a powerful tool that keeps you connected to your fitness journey. By routinely assessing your progress, celebrating victories, and making adjustments as needed, you create a more fulfilling and effective path for yourself. Embrace this practice and allow it to guide you toward achieving your fitness aspirations.

Celebrating Benchmarks

Celebrating your progress is an important part of any journey, especially in fitness. It's not just about finishing a race or achieving a certain weight; it's about appreciating everything you do along the way. Small celebrations are a great way to recognize your efforts and can take many forms. For example, if you have been consistent in your workouts for a week, treat yourself to a new piece of workout gear. This could be a new pair of shoes, a stylish gym bag, or even a fun water bottle that inspires you. When you surround yourself with things that make you happy, your motivation levels can increase, and working out can feel less like a chore.

Another way to celebrate progress is through food. After reaching a milestone—like completing a tough workout or hitting a personal best—enjoying a favorite healthy meal can be a rewarding experience. This could be something you make yourself, perhaps a colorful salad packed with your favorite veggies, or a satisfying smoothie that gives you a natural energy boost. The key is to make these celebrations feel special. They don't have to be lavish, but taking moments to celebrate what you've accomplished can keep your spirits high.

Each milestone along the way counts as an achievement, no matter how insignificant it might seem. For instance, finishing a week of consistent workouts is a significant step forward. It shows commitment and discipline, and this deserves recognition. Learning a new movement in Wall Pilates, which may feel challenging at first, is another success worth celebrating. It might take weeks to master, but when you finally do, it feels fantastic. Additionally, just feeling more energetic throughout the day is a transformation that should not be overlooked. This change impacts your quality of life and proves that the hard work is paying off.

When you take the time to celebrate these small victories, you create a ripple effect of positivity. Each celebration serves as a reminder of your capability and determination. This can lead to intrinsic motivation, which is the best kind because it comes from within. For example, knowing that you worked hard and completed a challenging workout will make you want to do it again. It motivates you to push your limits further because the reward is not just a treat but also a sense of pride in your accomplishments.

These moments of recognition don't just end with the celebration itself; they build on each other. When you acknowledge your efforts, you reinforce your commitment to your fitness goals. The next milestone you reach will feel even more rewarding because you've taken the time to celebrate previous achievements. It's a cycle of motivation that drives you forward.

Sharing your successes with friends or family can amplify the joy of these celebrations. When you tell someone about your latest achievement, it not only reinforces your success in your own mind, but it also invites others to celebrate with you. This can lead to a supportive environment where you all encourage one another. If you let your friends know that you've achieved a new goal, they might respond with applause, high-fives, or even plan a small celebration in your honor, such as a healthy dinner or a workout group. This shared experience can bring a sense of community to your fitness journey.

Remember, the progress you make in fitness is a path of continual growth and development. Every achievement, big or small, adds to your overall well-being. Embracing a mindset where you choose to celebrate can turn your fitness journey into an enjoyable and fulfilling experience. Instead of just focusing on the end result, find joy in the process, ensuring it feels enriching and rewarding.

Celebrating your fitness milestones helps maintain motivation. Whether it is through small personal rewards, enjoying a favorite meal, or sharing achievements with others, these practices keep the experience enjoyable. Every tiny success is worthy of recognition, helping you to cultivate a positive mindset and dedication to your journey. By finding moments of celebration throughout your process, you create a fulfilling and sustainable approach to fitness that goes beyond just physical changes.

Building on the Foundations We've Laid

In this chapter, we explored the foundational principles of designing entry-level to intermediate Wall Pilates programs with a focus on gradual progression. Emphasizing the importance of mastering basic movements such as wall planks, wall squats, and lateral wall slides, we underlined their role in building strength, flexibility, and confidence without overloading the body. By starting with minimal resistance and increasing intensity incrementally, participants can safely advance their skills while avoiding common injuries. This methodical approach ensures that both seniors and younger beginners can benefit from a structured and progressive fitness journey.

Next, we will address common injuries associated with physical activity, such as strains, sprains, and overuse injuries, setting the stage for a deeper exploration of preventive strategies. By focusing on Wall Pilates, we will not only emphasize the significance of strengthening muscles and enhancing flexibility but also highlight how individualizing routines can mitigate risks. This chapter will serve as a comprehensive resource for maintaining physical health and supporting rehabilitation, ensuring that practitioners are well-equipped to navigate their fitness journeys safely.

Chapter 8
Injury Prevention and Rehabilitation

I njury prevention and rehabilitation are crucial aspects of maintaining an active and fulfilling lifestyle, particularly for seniors and beginner fitness enthusiasts. Understanding how to effectively prevent injuries and recover from them ensures long-term health and physical well-being. With the growing popularity of Wall Pilates, individuals now have a versatile tool that combines strength-building, flexibility enhancement, and stability improvement to meet these needs. This chapter delves into how Wall Pilates can be employed as a preventive measure and a rehabilitation aid, offering practical insights and exercises tailored to different fitness levels and physical conditions.

As individuals incorporate Wall Pilates into their routines, it's vital to do so in a mindful manner. Focusing on proper form during each exercise minimizes the risk of injury. For example, one could begin with a basic side stretch while leaning against the wall. This exercise stretches the side muscles while providing a stable base for support. Practicing controlled movements helps build strength while reducing excessive strain on the body.

When it comes to rehabilitation, movement can play a key role in recovery. After an injury, many people might think they should avoid physical activity altogether. However, gentle exercises can ensure proper healing. For instance, those recovering from a sprained ankle might begin with low-impact movements, such as ankle circles or foot flexes, to promote strength and mobility without causing further damage.

Incorporating injury prevention techniques and proper rehabilitation practices into one's routine is essential for maintaining a healthy, active lifestyle. Wall Pilates serves as a versatile tool to support those processes, making fitness accessible and enjoyable for seniors and beginners alike. By understanding one's body and exercising mindfully, individuals can enjoy the benefits of a strong, flexible, and stable body while significantly reducing the risk of injuries.

Common Injuries and Preventive Measures

Injuries associated with physical activity are a significant concern for both seniors and beginner fitness enthusiasts. Common injuries often include strains, sprains, and overuse injuries. Strains occur when muscles or tendons are overstretched or torn, typically affecting the lower back, hamstrings, or shoulders. Sprains involve the stretching or tearing of ligaments around joints such as the ankle, knee, or wrist. Overuse injuries, including tendonitis and stress fractures, result from repetitive motion causing wear and tear on specific body parts. These injuries can deter individuals from maintaining an active lifestyle.

Wall Pilates offers effective strategies to mitigate these common injuries by focusing on exercises that build strength, improve flexibility, and enhance overall body stability. For instance, Wall Pilates incorporates isometric exercises where muscles contract without movement, providing resistance and promoting muscle endurance (Page, 2023). One such exercise is the wall sit, which engages the quadriceps, hamstrings, and glutes, strengthening the legs and reducing the risk of sprains during daily activities or workouts.

Enhancing flexibility is another critical aspect of injury prevention. Wall Pilates exercises like the elevated hip bridge help stretch the lower back and hamstrings, areas prone to strains. This stretching not only relieves tension but also enhances muscle elasticity, making the body more resilient to sudden movements that could cause injuries. Additionally, the static resistance provided by the wall helps maintain good form, ensuring that exercises target the correct muscle groups and minimize strain on joints.

Identifying personal risk factors is crucial in customizing a Wall Pilates routine to minimize injury risks effectively. Age is a significant factor; seniors may have reduced bone density and muscle mass, making them more susceptible to injuries. Beginner fitness enthusiasts might lack the necessary muscle support and balance, increasing their risk. Activity levels and existing conditions, such as arthritis or past injuries, also play a role. Understanding these factors helps tailor exercises to individual needs.

For seniors, low-impact exercises like leg raises, performed lying flat on the back with heels against the wall, are beneficial. They engage the core and improve lower body strength without putting undue stress on the joints. Beginners can start with simpler moves, gradually increasing intensity as their form and confidence improve. A mindful approach, listening to one's body, and modifying exercises as needed help prevent overexertion and ensure a safe progression in the workout routine.

Structuring a Wall Pilates practice to focus on minimizing injury risks requires thoughtful planning and consistency. Starting with a thorough warm-up is essential to prepare the muscles and joints for exercise. Gentle stretches and light movements help increase blood flow and flexibility. Incorporating a mix of strength-building and flexibility-enhancing exercises ensures a balanced workout. Exercises like incline push-ups, where the wall provides support, help build upper body strength while maintaining good form.

Alternating between different muscle groups during a workout prevents overuse of any single area. For example, pairing upper body exercises like wall push-ups with lower body moves like wall squats ensures comprehensive muscle engagement and balanced development. Cool-down periods with gentle stretching help relax the muscles and reduce post-exercise stiffness.

Consulting with a healthcare professional before starting the routine, especially for those with pre-existing conditions, ensures that the chosen exercises are safe and suitable. A personalized approach, respecting one's limitations while progressively challenging the body, promotes long-term adherence to the practice and reduces injury risks.

Rehabilitation Exercises for Recovery

Embarking on a rehabilitation journey post-injury can be a daunting task, but with careful planning and the right exercises, it becomes manageable and effective. For many, Wall Pilates offers a gentle yet potent method for aiding recovery, ensuring stability and strength are regained in a controlled manner.

Considerations When Starting Rehabilitation

Starting any rehabilitation program requires meticulous attention to detail, especially consulting healthcare providers. Before beginning Wall Pilates exercises, it is crucial to have an open discussion with your doctor or physical therapist. They can provide personalized advice tailored to your specific injury and overall health condition, ensuring that your rehabilitation plan aligns with medical recommendations. This foundational step forms the backbone of a safe and effective recovery process.

Understanding the body's signals is key. Pain, while often being part of recovery, should never be severe or sharp. It's essential to differentiate between discomfort due to muscle engagement and pain signaling potential harm. Being attuned to these bodily messages helps prevent exacerbating injuries and promotes a smoother path to recovery (Hardy, 2024).

Introducing Modified Wall Pilates Exercises

Once you have the green light from your healthcare provider, the next step is integrating modified Wall Pilates exercises into your routine. These exercises are designed to bolster stability and regain strength without overwhelming the body. Here are a few practical examples:

1. **Wall Roll-Downs** : Begin by standing with your back against the wall, feet shoulder-width apart. Slowly roll down, vertebra by vertebra, until your hands reach the ground. This movement aids in improving spine flexibility and core stability, crucial for maintaining a strong foundation during recovery (Stogdon, 2024).

1. **Wall Push-Ups** : Facing the wall, place your hands flat against it, slightly wider than shoulder-width. Perform a push-up by bending your elbows and leaning your body towards the wall, then push back to the starting position. This exercise strengthens the upper body muscles gently, building endurance without straining injured areas.

1. **Seated Leg Slides** : Sit with your back against the wall and legs extended. Slide one leg up, bending at the knee, then return to the extended position. Repeat with the other leg. This focuses on the core and lower body, enhancing muscle activation in a controlled environment.

1. **Wall Squats** : With your back against the wall, lower into a squat position, keeping your knees over your ankles. Hold this posture to strengthen your thighs and buttocks. Over time, aim to

extend the duration gradually as your strength and endurance improve.

These exercises are adaptable and can be scaled in intensity based on individual comfort levels and progress, forming a central part of a balanced rehabilitation regimen.

Strategies for Effectively Monitoring Progress During Rehabilitation

Tracking your progress throughout rehabilitation ensures you stay on the right track and make necessary adjustments promptly. Here are some effective strategies:

1. **Keeping a Recovery Journal** : Documenting your daily exercises, how you feel before and after workouts, pain levels, and any challenges encountered can provide valuable insights into your progress. Regular entries also facilitate communication with healthcare providers, allowing more precise guidance and adjustments to your rehabilitation plan.

1. **Setting Milestones** : Establish short-term and long-term goals that align with your overall recovery objectives. Short-term milestones might include completing a certain number of repetitions or holding a squat for a specified

duration. Long-term goals could focus on regaining full mobility or returning to pre-injury activity levels. Achieving these milestones provides motivation and concrete indicators of improvement.

1. **Regular Assessments by Professionals** : Periodic evaluations by your healthcare provider or a certified Pilates instructor can offer professional feedback on your technique and progression. They can identify areas needing improvement and suggest modifications to enhance efficiency and safety in your exercises.

1. **Using Technology** : Fitness apps and wearable devices can track various metrics such as heart rate, steps taken, and activity duration. Leveraging technology provides additional data points to monitor physical responses to exercises, helping refine your rehabilitation approach over time.

Tips on Gradually Increasing the Intensity of Wall Pilates Workouts as One Recovers

As the rehabilitation journey progresses, gradually increasing the intensity of Wall Pilates workouts ensures continued improvement while avoiding setbacks. The following tips can guide this transition:

1. **Listen to Your Body** : Always pay close attention to how your body reacts to increased intensity. Incremental changes should feel challenging but not overwhelming. If you experience significant discomfort, scale back and allow your body more time to adapt.

1. **Incremental Adjustments** : Start by adding small increments to your workout routine, such as increasing the number of repetitions or the duration of each exercise. For example, if you begin with five repetitions of wall push-ups, try adding one additional repetition every week.

1. **Incorporate Resistance Bands** : Introducing resistance bands adds another layer of challenge to your exercises. These flexible bands can be adjusted according to your strength level, providing customizable resistance that enhances muscle engagement and growth.

1. **Alternative Variations** : Enhance the complexity of basic exercises once they become easier. For instance, performing wall squats with a single leg or incorporating balance elements into

wall roll-downs can increase difficulty progressively, promoting strength and stability.

1. **Rest and Recovery** : Adequate rest between increased intensity sessions is vital. Muscles need time to repair and grow stronger, so ensure you incorporate rest days into your weekly routine. Hydration and nutrition also play pivotal roles in recovery, fueling your body for optimal performance and healing.

Strengthening Vulnerable Areas

Strengthening specific body areas that are often affected by injuries is crucial to reducing future risks and promoting overall wellness. By focusing on vulnerable regions such as the wrists, knees, and lower back, individuals can enhance their resilience and functionality in daily life. Wall Pilates offers a structured approach to achieving this goal through targeted exercises that build strength and stability.

The wrists are particularly susceptible to injury due to their involvement in various movements and weight-bearing activities. Exercises like Wall Push-ups help to strengthen the muscles around the wrist joints, providing greater support and reducing the risk of strains and sprains. This exercise not only targets the wrist muscles but also engages the shoulders and chest, contributing to overall upper body strength.

The knees are another common area of concern, especially for those who engage in physical activities or have a history of joint issues. Strengthening the quadriceps, hamstrings, and surrounding stabilizer muscles is essential for knee health. Wall Sits are effective for building knee strength. This exercise helps in improving muscle endurance and stability around the knee joints.

Lower back pain is a prevalent issue that can significantly impact quality of life. Targeting the deep postural muscles of the back, such as the multifidus, can provide relief and prevent future discomfort. One beneficial exercise is Pelvic Tilts against the wall. Lie on your back with your feet flat on the floor and knees bent. Press your lower back into the wall by engaging your abdominal muscles and tilting your pelvis upwards. Hold this position briefly before returning to neutral. Regular practice of Pelvic Tilts can enhance spinal stability and alleviate lower back pain.

Incorporating strength exercises that promote overall body strength while focusing on vulnerable areas is integral to a balanced routine. The Wall Bridge is a versatile exercise that targets multiple muscle groups, including the glutes, lower back, and hamstrings. Begin by lying on the floor with your feet resting on the wall at a 90-degree angle. Lift your hips off the ground, squeezing your glutes and maintaining a neutral spine. This movement not only strengthens the lower body but also supports core stability.

Monitoring strength improvement safely and effectively is essential to avoid overexertion and ensure progress. Setting realistic goals and tracking performance can motivate individuals and provide a clear sense of accomplishment. Using simple tools like resistance bands or light weights can help quantify strength gains. For instance, incorporating a resistance band into Wall Squats can add an extra challenge and allow for measurable progress. Begin with a lighter band and gradually increase resistance as strength improves.

It's important to listen to your body and recognize the signs of fatigue or discomfort. Rest and recovery are crucial components of any fitness regimen, allowing muscles to repair and grow stronger. Consulting with a healthcare provider or a certified Pilates instructor can provide personalized guidance and modifications based on individual needs and limitations (Archer Pilates, 2018).

Performing regular self-assessments can also be valuable. Simple tests such as holding a Wall Sit for a longer duration or adding more repetitions to Wall Push-ups can indicate improvements in strength and endurance. Keeping a fitness journal to record these assessments, along with any changes in how exercises feel, can offer insights into progress and areas that might need additional focus.

Moving Forward with Confidence

This chapter has explored the effectiveness of Wall Pilates in preventing injuries and aiding rehabilitation. By focusing on exercises that build strength, enhance flexibility, and improve overall stability, Wall Pilates helps mitigate common injuries like strains, sprains, and overuse injuries. Specific techniques such as wall sits, elevated hip bridges, and incline push-ups offer targeted benefits to vulnerable areas, ensuring a balanced approach to physical health. Understanding individual risk factors and customizing workouts based on age, fitness level, and existing conditions further enhances safety and efficacy.

For those recovering from injuries, integrating Wall Pilates into a rehabilitation routine proves beneficial. Modified exercises like wall roll-downs, wall push-ups, and seated leg slides support gradual recovery by strengthening muscles without overwhelming the body. Monitoring progress through keeping a recovery journal, setting milestones, and using technology ensures a well-rounded rehabilitation process. Consulting healthcare professionals for personalized advice and gradually increasing exercise intensity can lead to sustained improvements in strength and flexibility. Ultimately, consistent practice of Wall Pilates fosters long-term physical health and resilience.

Building on this, we now turn our attention to practical implementation. The next chapter will guide readers on how to seamlessly integrate Wall Pilates into different parts of their day, transforming it into a natural and enjoyable aspect of their routines. We will explore strategies that cater to various lifestyles, ensuring that the benefits of Wall Pilates extend beyond the studio and into everyday life. This transition emphasizes the importance of consistency and adaptability in practice, setting the stage for readers to cultivate a sustainable relationship with Wall Pilates as a cherished part of their daily regimen.

Chapter 9
Integrating Wall Pilates into Daily Life

I ntegrating Wall Pilates into daily life can be a rewarding endeavor that enhances both physical and mental well-being. By finding creative ways to incorporate these exercises into everyday routines, individuals of all ages and fitness levels can experience the numerous benefits of consistent practice. Whether you are looking to maintain functional strength as you age or simply seeking an effective way to start a new fitness habit, Wall Pilates offers a versatile solution that fits seamlessly into even the busiest of schedules.

Quick Routines for Busy Schedules

Incorporating short Wall Pilates routines into daily life doesn't have to be overwhelming. Even amidst a hectic schedule, finding pockets of time for these exercises can offer immense benefits. Here's how you can seamlessly weave Wall Pilates into your day.

5-Minute Morning Wake-Up

Starting your day with a quick 5-minute Wall Pilates routine can ignite your body and prepare it for the day ahead. Simple stretches are a great way to awaken your core and enhance flexibility. Begin by standing against the wall, ensuring your feet are hip-width apart. Slowly raise your arms over your head while inhaling deeply. As you exhale, roll down through your spine, trying to touch your toes or reaching as far as comfortable. This gentle stretch helps release any tension accumulated overnight and kick-starts your metabolism.

Continuing with core engagement, you can perform wall squats. Stand with your back against the wall, slide down into a squat position as if sitting on an invisible chair, hold for a few seconds, then slowly rise up. This move not only activates the major muscle groups but also improves your balance and posture.

Another effective exercise is the wall bridge. Lie on your back with your feet placed firmly against the wall, knees bent at 90 degrees. Lift your hips towards the ceiling while squeezing your glutes, hold for a breath, and lower back down. These moves, performed consistently, can set a positive tone for the rest of your day.

Lunchtime Wall Break

For those who struggle to find workout time during the workday, fitting a Wall Pilates routine into your lunch hour can be a game-changer. Techniques such as wall push-ups or seated chair stretches can be done in confined spaces, focusing on posture and productivity enhancement.

Start with wall push-ups to engage your upper body. Place your hands on the wall at shoulder height and width, walk your feet back until you're leaning in at an angle. Slowly bend your elbows, bringing your chest towards the wall, and then push back to start. This exercise strengthens the arms and shoulders while requiring minimal space.

Seated chair stretches are another excellent option. While seated, cross one leg over the other knee and gently press down on your knee to deepen the stretch, switching sides after a few breaths. This stretch aids in opening the hips and relieving lower back tension, vital for those spending long hours at a desk.

Using a wall for support, you can perform calf raises. Stand facing the wall with your hands resting on it for balance. Raise onto your tiptoes, hold for a moment, then lower back down. This simple move engages the calves and enhances circulation, providing a midday energy boost that can improve focus and productivity.

Evening Wind Down

As the day winds down, a calming evening routine involving Wall Pilates can aid relaxation and mindfulness. Linking this practice with bedtime preparations ensures consistency and helps transition from the day's hustle to a state of restfulness.

Begin with wall-supported stretches. Sit with your back against the wall, legs extended straight out. Slowly reach forward, aiming to touch your toes, allowing your back to gently round over. This forward fold releases tension in the back and hamstrings, promoting relaxation.

Next, try the wall roll-down. Stand a few inches away from the wall, back facing it. Starting from your neck, gradually roll down vertebra by vertebra, letting your arms hang loose. Roll back up just as slowly. This controlled movement encourages mindfulness and a heightened awareness of your body's sensations.

Incorporating gentle breathing exercises can further enhance the winding-down process. Standing with your back against the wall, close your eyes, take deep breaths, and focus on the rise and fall of your abdomen. This practice not only calms the mind but also prepares your body for restful sleep.

Weekend Mini-Sessions

Weekends offer more flexibility, making them ideal for slightly longer Wall Pilates workouts. These mini-sessions can keep your motivation high and allow for the introduction of new routines. Planning a 20-minute session on Saturday mornings, for instance, can set a healthy tone for the entire weekend.

Start with exercises like wall sit-and-reach. Position yourself in a wall sit, where your thighs are parallel to the ground, and alternate reaching one arm over your head while maintaining the squat position. This combination of stability and mobility enhances both strength and flexibility.

Another beneficial exercise is the single-leg wall squat. Standing with your back against the wall, lift one leg, keeping it straight, and squat down on the supporting leg. Return to standing and switch sides. This variation challenges your balance and core strength, adding a new dimension to your routine.

Community engagement can also be incorporated on weekends. Joining a local Wall Pilates class or participating in online sessions can provide a sense of community and accountability. This social aspect can make the practice more enjoyable and sustainable, encouraging you to stick with it in the long run. For example, many communities offer outdoor classes, which bring the added benefit of fresh air and nature's relaxing ambiance.

Dedicating time on weekends to learn new exercises or variations can prevent your routine from becoming monotonous. Exploring different movements keeps you engaged and continuously challenges your body, promoting steady progress.

Blending Wall Pilates with Other Activities

Incorporating Wall Pilates into daily life can be an enriching experience, especially when combined with other physical activities. This approach not only keeps the practice dynamic but also ensures that it fits seamlessly into various aspects of one's routine without feeling like a chore. By blending Wall Pilates with activities such as walking, family exercises, other fitness classes, and community events, practitioners can experience a holistic enhancement in their physical and mental well-being.

Practicing Mindful Movement During Walks

Walking is a very easy way to add movement to your daily life. When you walk, you can turn this simple activity into something more meaningful by using principles from Pilates. Pilates focuses on posture awareness and controlled breathing, which can make your walks not just about getting from one place to another, but also about connecting with your body and mind. This transformation begins with paying careful attention to how you hold your body while you walk.

To start, let's think about your posture. Good posture is essential for walking in a way that keeps your body safe and feeling good. First, make sure your spine is straight. An easy way to do this is to stand tall before you start walking. Imagine there is a string pulling you up from the top of your head. Keep your shoulders relaxed and away from your ears, which can help prevent any shoulder tension. Next, engage your core. This means tightening your stomach muscles a little, which helps support your back and keeps your body balanced as you walk. Keeping good alignment while walking is something that Pilates teaches, and following this principle helps improve how your body moves. It can also help you avoid injuries, making your walking experience more pleasurable and safer.

Another important part of Pilates is how you breathe. Controlled breathing can make a big difference in how you feel while walking. While you are walking, try to practice deep breathing. This is often referred to as diaphragmatic breathing. To do this, inhale deeply through your nose. When you breathe in, focus on letting your abdomen expand naturally. This allows for more air to fill your lungs. After a good inhalation, exhale slowly through your mouth. This not only helps increase the oxygen flowing in your body but also has a calming effect on your mind. When you breathe this way, it helps you feel more centered and aware of what's happening in your body.

Combining these mindful practices with your walks makes the experience more beneficial. Instead of just moving your legs, you begin to make each step count. By focusing on your posture and breathing, you are not only exercising your body but also engaging your mind. This means that every step you take can be a reminder to check in with yourself, your body, and your breath.

As you walk, try to notice the world around you as well. Look at the colors of the trees and the sky. Listen to the sounds, like birds chirping or leaves rustling in the wind. Allowing your mind to be aware of your surroundings while practicing mindful movement can enrich your experience. This connection to your environment can enhance your walks, making them feel more rewarding.

Practicing mindful movement while walking helps develop a routine that you can look forward to. Begin by choosing a time of day that works best for you. Some people prefer mornings to start their day refreshed, while others might enjoy a peaceful walk in the evening to wind down. Whatever time you choose, set it aside regularly to make walking a part of your routine.

After making walking a regular part of your life, you'll likely start to notice the benefits. You may feel more energetic throughout the day. Your body may feel more aligned and less tense. The time you spend in nature or on the streets can help enhance your mood. The combination of exercise and mindful observation can also lead to clearer thinking.

For some days, if you prefer a change, consider mixing up your route. Walking in new places can spark excitement and curiosity. Explore different parks or neighborhoods and notice how each setting has a unique vibe. Every new location brings different sights, sounds, and smells that can enrich your experience.

In addition to these simple practices, try to challenge yourself gradually. If you usually walk for 20 minutes, consider extending that time to 30 minutes. You might also try adding an incline, like a small hill. As you become more comfortable and confident in your movement, you can explore different speeds or intervals. Perhaps try walking faster for a minute, then slowing down for another. This kind of varied movement can keep walks engaging while continuing to honor the mindfulness approach Pilates offers.

Creating a mindful walking routine based on Pilates principles can be fulfilling. Not only can it enhance your physical well-being, but it also cultivates a sense of mindfulness that can translate into other areas of your life. Each walk becomes a chance to connect deeply with yourself, your breath, and the world around you. Ultimately, this practice supports overall health, peace of mind, and a more meaningful daily routine.

Making Wall Pilates a Family-Friendly Exercise

Engaging in physical activities with family members can create enjoyable moments and help everyone stay healthy. One great way to do this is by making Wall Pilates a family-friendly exercise. Wall Pilates can be an effective way for families to work together towards better health. When everyone takes part, the atmosphere becomes lively and engaging. It promotes health and well-being for all ages, making it a perfect choice for family activities.

One of the simplest ways to start is by doing wall-supported exercises. For example, wall squats are easy and can be done by anyone. You can turn wall squats into a fun family challenge. Everyone can take turns attempting to hold the squat for a certain amount of time. This challenge not only promotes physical activity but also creates laughter and joy as family members cheer each other on. Another simple exercise is the wall arm stretch. While stretching, family members can count aloud or reach for a special point on the wall, making it more interactive and fun.

For younger children, adding playful elements can make Wall Pilates even more enjoyable. For instance, while doing exercises, you could count reps together out loud. This can be turned into a game where children can guess the number of squats before you finish counting. You could also make it exciting by pretending to reach for imaginary objects. For example, while stretching, everyone can reach for invisible apples on the wall. Balancing games can be a hit too, such as seeing who can keep their balance longer against the wall. These activities not only make exercising enjoyable but also help children learn to be active in a fun way.

When involving seniors in Wall Pilates, it's essential to make sure everyone feels safe and comfortable. Modifications can make a big difference. For example, using a chair for support during certain exercises can ensure that seniors can join in without feeling unsteady. Simple wall pushes or gentle stretches can be performed with the support of a chair, ensuring that everyone can participate regardless of their fitness level. It just takes a little creativity to adapt the exercises so that they fit the needs of every age group.

The shared experience of doing these exercises together also builds motivation and accountability among family members. When everyone is working towards a common goal, it becomes easier to stick with a routine. Setting specific times during the week for family Pilates sessions can create a sense of commitment. You might choose to exercise every Saturday morning or Wednesday evening. These dedicated times can quickly turn into cherished family traditions, enhancing both health and family ties.

Modeling physical activity is an excellent way to set a positive example for children. When children see their parents or relatives getting involved in exercise, they are more likely to follow suit. This modeling helps children understand the importance of staying active. It promotes healthy habits that can last a lifetime. For instance, even if children see their parents doing stretches or enjoying exercise, they may be inspired to do it themselves. Grabbing a mat and exercising alongside family members can create a warm environment for fitness.

As family members engage in Wall Pilates, having a fun, light-hearted atmosphere can be crucial. Leaning on a wall to hold spinal stretches or lunges while chatting with one another can create a sense of connection and joy. When you laugh and enjoy yourselves, the pressure of exercise tends to lessen. Relaxed moments can help family members feel good about themselves and boost their confidence. This, in turn, can lead to healthier relationships with exercise.

In addition to fun exercises, it's also important to talk about health and fitness together. Family members can discuss the benefits of being active and how it helps everyone feel better physically and mentally. Make it a point to share stories about how exercise has changed your day, improved your mood, or increased your energy. This dialogue can inspire everyone to think positively about the exercise they do together.

Another great way to keep the family engaged is by planning special event days around your Wall Pilates sessions. For instance, you could have a "Fitness Family Day" where everyone gets to pick their favorite mini-exercise to do against the wall. Perhaps one family member loves to do jumping jacks while wall-sitting at the same time. Another might enjoy trying different stretches. A family day can lead to everyone sharing ideas and learning new exercises from each other.

Lastly, celebrating small achievements is essential in making Wall Pilates a family-friendly exercise. You can recognize milestones, such as completing a particular number of sessions or improving form and balance. A simple clap, high-five, or even a family award like a homemade trophy or certificate can make family members feel appreciated and motivated to continue. Fun and encouragement go hand in hand with exercise, creating a fantastic foundation for lifelong fitness practices.

Making Wall Pilates a family-friendly exercise requires creativity, interaction, and support. By embracing everyone's strengths and interests, Wall Pilates can easily fit into family life. Keeping it fun, safe, and engaging will ensure that everyone in the family benefits. Encourage active participation, celebrate achievements, and share experiences. All these elements can turn Wall Pilates into a wholesome family activity that enriches both health and connections.

Combining Pilates with Other Fitness Classes

Variety in exercise routines is important for maintaining interest and motivation. When we incorporate different types of exercise, we can reduce boredom and increase our overall fitness. One exciting way to achieve this is by combining Wall Pilates with other fitness classes. By mixing these classes, you can create a well-rounded workout that focuses on flexibility, balance, and strength. Understanding the benefits of each type of exercise can help you see how they complement each other.

The Role of Yoga

Yoga is a practice that emphasizes stretching, mindfulness, and breath control. These elements are beneficial for your body and mind. When we practice yoga, we learn to connect our movements with our breath. This helps in relaxing and focusing. Wall Pilates, on the other hand, primarily targets the core muscles and works on stability. By adding yoga to your routine, you can enhance your understanding of body mechanics. This means you will become more aware of how different parts of your body interact during movement. For beginners, starting with simple yoga poses like downward dog or child's pose can be a great introduction. As your flexibility improves, you can gradually move to more complex poses. This process not only helps prevent injuries but also aids in improving functional movement patterns in daily activities.

Bringing Dance into the Mix

Dance classes add a different dimension to your fitness routine. They focus on rhythm, coordination, and the fluidity of movement. When you include dance with Wall Pilates, you introduce an exciting element of grace and agility to your workouts. The combination of dance and Pilates allows your body to move in new and creative ways. For instance, consider taking a jazz or ballet class alongside Pilates.

These styles will encourage you to explore the rhythm in your movements and develop better coordination. Engaging in dance also keeps your heart rate up, which is beneficial for cardiovascular health.

The Fusion of Practices

Integrating dance with Wall Pilates not only keeps your exercise routine enjoyable but also provides numerous physical benefits. This mix helps improve muscle tone and endurance. As you practice both forms of exercise, you will notice increased strength in your core and improved overall body control. It can also boost mental clarity, as rhythmic movements in dance engage the brain in different ways. To get started, you might want to try a class that blends Pilates and dance. Many local studios offer hybrid classes where you can experience the benefits of both exercises in one session. By participating in these classes, you will be guided by trained instructors who can help you learn the correct techniques and ensure you stay safe while exercising.

Exploration of Options

The fitness world is evolving, and many studios now offer a variety of classes that combine elements from different disciplines, including Pilates, yoga, and dance. These hybrid classes provide a unique opportunity to explore how each form of exercise can support and enhance the others. When looking for a class, it's helpful to read reviews or ask around in your community. Finding the right fit can make a big difference in your fitness journey. Consider trying out different classes to discover what you enjoy the most. The variety keeps you engaged and motivated to reach your fitness goals.

Making exercise a fun and varied experience can lead to more sustained commitment. By exploring different options and combinations, you can personalize your fitness routine to best suit your interests and needs. Whether you prefer the calm and focus of yoga, the dynamic movements of dance, or the core-strengthening benefits of Pilates, there is something out there for everyone. This personalized approach can lead to better results and a greater enjoyment of the activities you choose to participate in.

Participating in Community Events or Organizing Local Wall Pilates Sessions

Engaging in community events or setting up local Wall Pilates sessions can boost motivation for physical activity. When people participate in community fitness activities, they create a network of support with others who share similar health goals. This communal spirit can significantly enhance the motivation to stay active. For example, by attending a fitness event in your area, you may find people who are at different fitness levels. This provides a chance for everyone to share their experiences and learn from one another, making the journey to better health feel less lonely.

Organizing a Wall Pilates session in a park or community center is a great way to bring people together. To start, you might want to team up with a local fitness instructor. An experienced instructor can lead the sessions and provide valuable insights to participants. This not only enhances the quality of the session, but it also offers a safe space for beginners to learn proper techniques. Promoting these activities is essential to gathering participants. You can easily reach out to people through social media platforms, local community boards, or newsletters to spread the word. Effective promotion can ensure that interested individuals know when and where the sessions will take place.

Creating a welcoming environment can make these events even more enjoyable. Consider setting up the session in an inviting location, where attendees can feel comfortable and relaxed. Adding light refreshments or playing soft music can help create a friendly atmosphere that encourages people to interact and bond. The focus should be on fostering camaraderie among participants, which can lead to lasting friendships and support systems. When individuals feel they are part of a community, they are more likely to stay committed to their fitness journeys.

Another motivating idea is to initiate public fitness challenges. For instance, a 30-day Wall Pilates challenge can engage many people at once. Participants can keep track of their progress, perhaps using a shared online platform to post updates and share their achievements. Celebrating milestones together can create a sense of achievement among the group. When participants see how others are progressing, it can inspire them to push themselves further. This collective effort makes each individual feel supported and accountable.

Social media can also play a vital role in engaging the community. Creating a dedicated group for participants to share tips, success stories, and even struggles can strengthen bonds. By checking in regularly and encouraging each other, individuals can maintain their motivation to stick to their fitness goals. People often appreciate the chance to share their progress, and seeing others actively engaged can serve as positive reinforcement.

It's also important to consider how participants can engage at varying skill levels. Taking this into account allows for a more inclusive environment, where everyone can learn and grow at their own pace. Offering modifications for different skill levels during a Wall Pilates session ensures that no one feels left out. Newcomers may appreciate guidance on technique, while more experienced attendees can be challenged with advanced movements. This adaptability can help all participants benefit from the session.

When organizing these events, ensure that there is something for everyone. Besides the Wall Pilates sessions, consider including additional activities related to fitness and well-being. Workshops on nutrition, mental health, or recovery techniques can offer participants a well-rounded experience and increase engagement. By diversifying the offerings, participants may be more inclined to attend regularly. This helps solidify the sense of community, as individuals gather not only for physical exercise but also to learn and grow together.

Engaging with local businesses can also help enhance community events. Local health food stores or cafes might be interested in sponsoring or joining in on these events. They could provide snacks or goodies that align with health goals. Such partnerships can introduce participants to new healthy options and build a sense of local pride. When communities come together in this way, it strengthens the network of support, and everyone benefits from one another's contributions.

Seeking feedback from participants after each event can improve future sessions. Knowing what others liked or what they thought could be better allows you to tailor future events more effectively. It shows participants that their opinions matter and that their experiences shape the offerings in the community. Consistent improvement can keep the community vibrant and engaging, helping individuals feel more inclined to be involved.

Lastly, creating a sense of routine can help foster commitment to fitness activities. Regularly scheduled Wall Pilates sessions at the same time each week allow participants to carve out that time in their schedules. Just like any other important appointment, making time for fitness can lead to long-term habits. Over time, attendees are likely to see improvements in their strength, flexibility, and overall well-being, reinforcing the efforts they put into participating and engaging with the community.

Overall, engaging in community fitness events like Wall Pilates can create an enriching and supportive environment. By collaborating with local instructors, promoting activities effectively, and ensuring an inclusive atmosphere for all skill levels, these initiatives help improve health collectively. By using social media and engaging with local businesses, the network of support can continue to grow. The journey towards better health becomes much more enjoyable when it is shared with others, making the experience memorable and rewarding for everyone involved.

Creating a Home Practice Environment

Creating a conducive home environment for practicing Wall Pilates is paramount in ensuring that you can seamlessly integrate this beneficial exercise into your daily life. This section will guide you through the essentials of setting up your space, selecting the right tools, maintaining a consistent schedule, and involving family members in your practice.

First and foremost, selecting and optimizing a quiet, clutter-free space is crucial for effective Wall Pilates practice. A serene environment devoid of distractions allows better focus on the exercises. Look for a spot in your home that has an uncluttered wall with enough open floor space to move comfortably. Make sure the area promotes relaxation by incorporating personal touches that inspire motivation, such as plants, calming artwork, or even a small fountain. These elements can create a soothing atmosphere, making your practice more enjoyable and grounding.

Once you've identified your practice space, gathering the necessary tools is the next step. Essential equipment like a high-quality Pilates mat provides comfort and stability during exercises. Mats with good cushioning protect your joints and enhance your overall experience, particularly important for seniors looking to maintain functional strength. Blocks and straps are also recommended as they help in modifying exercises to accommodate different fitness levels, ensuring safety and efficacy. Including resistance bands and foam rollers can add variety to your workouts, enabling you to target different muscle groups and prevent monotony.

Visual aids such as posters or videos can be incredibly helpful, especially for beginners. Posters illustrating key exercises can guide you through your routines when you're practicing alone, ensuring correct form and technique. Videos offer the advantage of real-time demonstration, which can be particularly useful if you prefer a guided session over memorized routines. Having these aids readily visible and accessible in your practice space can make your sessions more structured and efficient (Oravisto, 2023).

To build consistency in your Wall Pilates routine, creating a visible schedule within your practice area is highly beneficial. A physical calendar or planner placed on the wall where you practice can serve as a constant reminder and motivator. Marking out specific times dedicated to your Pilates sessions helps establish a routine that feels natural and unforced. Consider scheduling sessions at similar times each day to build a habit, whether it's early morning to start your day energized or evenings to wind down. Seasonal variations can also keep your practice engaging. For example, lighter routines in summer months focusing on stretching and core work can be followed by more strengthening exercises in the winter. The dynamic shift in routines not only keeps things exciting but also ensures balanced development of strength and flexibility year-round.

Personalizing your Pilates space by adding elements that resonate with you and your family can further enhance your commitment to regular practice. Inspirational quotes, family photos, or even a sound system for your favorite music playlists can make the space uniquely yours. These personal touches transform the practice area into a welcoming and motivating retreat, rather than just another corner of your home.

Finally, investing in a well-thought-out setup pays dividends in terms of convenience and effectiveness. With a designated area equipped with necessary tools and visual aids, following a routine becomes less of a chore and more of a ritual you look forward to. Moreover, involving your family brings additional joy and satisfaction, reinforcing the importance of consistent practice.

Final Insights

In this chapter, we have explored various strategies for integrating Wall Pilates into daily routines, providing practical examples tailored to different times of the day. Starting with a morning wake-up routine, and extending through midday breaks, evening wind-downs, and weekend mini-sessions, these practices are designed to fit seamlessly into busy schedules. By emphasizing simple yet effective exercises, individuals can gradually build strength, flexibility, and mindfulness without feeling overwhelmed.

The key takeaway is the importance of consistency and adaptability in your Wall Pilates practice. Even short sessions can yield significant benefits when performed regularly. Whether you are a senior looking to maintain functional strength or a beginner seeking an accessible fitness routine, these guidelines offer a flexible approach to staying active. Incorporating Wall Pilates into your daily activities not only promotes physical health but also enhances overall well-being, making it a valuable addition to any lifestyle.

As we conclude this chapter and explore the practical integration of Wall Pilates into our daily routines, it's essential to recognize that the journey of wellness is often enriched by community engagement. Imagine stepping into a vibrant network of like-minded individuals who share your passion for health and fitness—this is the heart of our next chapter. Here, we will delve into the myriad ways to connect with fellow Wall Pilates enthusiasts. By fostering these connections, not only can we enhance our practice, but we can also create a supportive environment that encourages collective growth and camaraderie in our Wall Pilates journey.

Chapter 10
Building a Supportive Community

Building a supportive community is necessary for anyone engaged in Wall Pilates. Whether through local classes or online platforms, being part of a group offers motivation and accountability that can significantly enhance your practice. The sense of camaraderie and shared goals helps to keep individuals motivated and committed, ensuring they continue to derive the full benefits of Wall Pilates.

Having a supportive community means having access to shared experiences and knowledge. When individuals come together, they exchange tips about techniques, share progress, and celebrate small victories. This collective wisdom can help newcomers avoid common pitfalls and make their practice more effective. Having someone to ask questions helps deepen understanding. It encourages learning, which is essential in any physical practice.

Encouragement plays a huge role. A simple 'you can do it' from a fellow participant can give someone the push they need to try a challenging pose or to make it through a tough class. This kind of support can lead to breakthroughs that individuals might not achieve on their own. It's really motivating to see friends progress, and it can inspire personal growth. Being in a community means you can lift each other up, creating an uplifting environment that fosters improvement and enjoyment.

Accountability is another major benefit of community involvement. When others are invested in your journey, you're less likely to skip a session or lose focus. Setting goals together and checking in on each other's progress creates a sense of commitment. Individuals can encourage one another to stay on track, which is especially helpful when motivation wanes. The group dynamic can help ensure everyone shows up and gives their best effort, leading to greater overall success.

Sharing challenges can also strengthen bonds within the community. Wall Pilates can be difficult, and everyone faces hurdles along their journey. When members talk about their struggles, it normalizes those feelings and reminds everyone they're not alone. The community becomes a safe space for sharing fears and concerns. This shared understanding creates deeper connections, fostering friendships that go beyond just the workouts. It's comforting to know that there's a group of people who truly understand the ups and downs of the practice.

Regular group classes or online sessions can also help create routines. Consistency is key in any fitness regimen and being part of a community can help establish that. Scheduled classes provide an easy way to commit to your practice. Members may coordinate their schedules or motivate each other to show up, which instills discipline. Over time, this routine becomes part of daily life, enhancing both physical and mental well-being.

Having a diverse community enriches the experience. Different perspectives and backgrounds contribute to a richer understanding of Wall Pilates. People bring unique styles, insights, and techniques that can teach others something new. This diversity can also make the workouts more fun, as individuals share different forms of music, equipment, and exercises. Variety keeps the practice engaging and helps prevent monotony from settling in.

Sharing resources is another significant advantage. In a supportive community, participants often share recommendations for classes, instructors, or online resources. This can lead to discovering new techniques or classes that align well with personal goals. The ability to benefit from others' research and experiences can save time and enhance one's practice. Having knowledgeable members improves the quality of the community, creating a valuable asset for everyone involved.

Group discussions about principles of Wall Pilates can further deepen understanding. Conversations about alignment, breath, and flow can clarify the practice's foundations. These discussions provide insights into how to maximize benefits and prevent injuries. Knowledge shared within the community boosts confidence in performing movements correctly and safely. Learning from one another helps reinforce the overall commitment to the practice.

Access to different levels of expertise also transforms the community. Beginners can seek guidance from advanced members, while experienced practitioners can benefit from fresh perspectives. This mentorship dynamic fosters an environment of growth. As members challenge one another, everyone has the opportunity to improve at their own pace. A supportive community promotes learning while encouraging growth, showcasing the beauty of shared knowledge and collective upliftment.

Social gatherings outside of classes can help strengthen these bonds. Sharing a meal or participating in social events allows members to connect on a personal level. These interactions foster a sense of belonging and make it easier to approach one another during class. Building friendships outside of workouts encourages open communication and further enhances motivation. When people care about each other, they become more invested in everyone's success.

Feeling comfortable in a community encourages vulnerability. Sharing fears or struggles can be intimidating, but having a supportive group makes it easier. Those who feel comfortable expressing themselves can receive constructive feedback, enhancing their practice. The environment created by the community encourages individuals to be open and honest, leading to growth. Vulnerability allows for personal connection, strengthening relationships among members.

Community also offers opportunities for collaboration. Members can partner up during exercises, providing additional support and feedback in real-time. Working together helps individuals learn from one another and motivates them to push beyond their limits. This collaborative practice creates a dynamic environment where everyone can grow, learn, and improve.

Personal stories of transformation can serve as powerful motivators. Members sharing their journeys often inspire others to take that first step. Hearing about someone conquering challenges or overcoming setbacks can ignite a spark in others and instill hope. These narratives create a sense of possibility and emphasize the power of perseverance. Personal connections through storytelling enhance the community dynamic, as individuals relate to one another's struggles and achievements.

In the end, a supportive community creates a nurturing environment where each member can thrive. When individuals share their experiences, encourage each other, and commit to collective growth, the entire group flourishes. Being part of such a community enriches the Wall Pilates experience and ensures that everyone enjoys the journey towards their personal goals.

Finding Local or Online Support Groups

Engaging in Wall Pilates can be a transformative experience, especially when you are part of a supportive community. These communities provide motivation, accountability, and an invaluable sense of belonging. Here's how you can tap into these networks to enrich your Wall Pilates journey.

Local Wall Pilates Classes and Workshops

Attending local Wall Pilates classes is a fantastic way to immerse yourself in this exercise practice. It allows you to not only focus on your fitness but also to connect with other people who have similar fitness goals. When you participate in these classes, you often find a sense of community. This community is built on a shared interest in improving health and fitness. The camaraderie that grows in a class setting is incredible. It helps motivate you to attend regularly. Having a group of fellow practitioners cheering you on can significantly boost your moral support.

Having local instructors is another bonus. They provide critical feedback in real time. This immediate support helps you refine your technique and avoids potential injuries. When instructors are close by, they can correct your posture and suggest modifications suited for your level. This hands-on support is invaluable, especially if you're just starting out with Wall Pilates.

If you want to find local Wall Pilates classes, there are a few simple steps to follow. First, consider searching through online directories that list various fitness classes in your area. Websites and apps dedicated to exercise and fitness often have detailed information about local classes, including times, locations, and even reviews. You might also want to ask friends or family for recommendations. If they have had positive experiences with a particular instructor or studio, that can lead you to a welcoming environment.

Visiting your local gym or fitness center is another good step. Many gyms have bulletin boards where they post information about local classes. You can often find flyers or schedules that detail when Wall Pilates classes are offered. Staff members at these gyms can also point you in the right direction. They are typically knowledgeable about what classes would suit beginners or those looking to enhance their skills.

Another great option is to look for beginner-friendly workshops. Many studios offer special sessions designed for those who are new to Wall Pilates. These workshops usually focus on teaching basic techniques while ensuring participants feel supported. They often take the time to go over foundational movements and give participants a chance to practice in a relaxed setting. This focus on beginner skills allows participants to gain confidence before moving on to more advanced classes.

Remember that in any exercise practice, the most important aspect is to listen to your body. Pilates can be both challenging and accessible, depending on your current fitness level. As you join different classes, you will likely learn how to modify moves to suit your own abilities and limitations. Instructors typically advocate for moving at your own pace, which is helpful. It's not just about doing an exercise correctly; it's about doing what feels right for you.

As you attend classes, do not hesitate to ask questions. Instructors are there to help, and they welcome inquiries. Whether it's about a specific pose or how to adjust your form, an open dialogue can enhance your learning experience. Engaging with your instructor can also help solidify your understanding, making the practice more fulfilling.

If you are considering joining local Wall Pilates classes, know that you're making a great choice for your health and social well-being. You'll learn new skills, meet supportive fellow practitioners, and receive guidance from knowledgeable instructors. Taking that first step can lead to a rewarding journey in fitness and self-discovery.

Online Platforms and Social Media Groups

For many people, attending in-person workouts can be difficult. This is where online platforms come in. They offer a wonderful alternative for those who want to participate in Pilates from the comfort of their own homes. These virtual spaces allow anyone interested in Pilates to join groups that focus specifically on this form of exercise. With the rise of technology, you can now find communities dedicated to Pilates on popular platforms like YouTube, Facebook, and other fitness forums. This makes it easier for individuals to access Pilates practices no matter where they are or what their daily schedules look like.

One of the key advantages of joining an online Pilates community is how flexible it can be. People have busy lives—some are juggling jobs, family duties, or other commitments. Participating in an online group allows for the choice of when and how much you want to engage. You can pick a time that suits you to watch workout videos, participate in discussions, or ask questions. This accessibility ensures that anyone, regardless of their location, can benefit from Pilates. If you live in a place where in-person classes are not available, online platforms eliminate that barrier.

When you decide to join an online Wall Pilates community, the first step is to find the right groups. On social media platforms, you can search for keywords or hashtags related to Wall Pilates. For example, using hashtags like #WallPilates or #PilatesCommunity can help you discover groups that suit your interests. Take the time to join several of these groups to broaden your exposure to different instructors and practices. By being part of multiple groups, you get the chance to learn from various perspectives and find what resonates with you the most.

Once you find the group that fits your needs, it is important to participate actively. Engagement is crucial in any community. You can start by sharing your experiences and insights about your Pilates journey. You might discuss the challenges you face, your progress, or even the routines that you enjoy. This exchange of ideas not only enriches your own experience but also contributes positively to the group. When you connect with others, it can inspire you and motivate you to keep going.

Another way to enhance your online Pilates experience is by taking part in events organized by the community. Online challenges, for instance, can be a great way to stay committed. These challenges often encourage participants to set goals over a specific period, such as 30 days of daily Pilates routines. By participating, you establish a sense of accountability. When you know there are others working alongside you, you may be more likely to stick to your goals. This collective effort can create a supportive environment that fosters growth and progress.

In addition to challenges, many communities also organize live-streamed classes. These sessions allow you to follow along with an instructor in real-time. This interaction can help you stay on track and develop a routine. There's something motivating about working out together, even if it's all happening through a screen. You can ask questions on-the-spot or get instant feedback, which can be very beneficial for your practice.

Remember, the essence of an online community lies in consistent interaction. The more you engage with others, the more you will gain from the experience. Regular contributions to discussions help you stay connected. By sharing your milestones, whether they are big or small, you contribute to a culture of encouragement. Celebrating your achievements, even those that seem minor, can uplift not just yourself but also those around you.

Offering encouragement to fellow members can amplify the sense of community. Everyone in the group is on their own journey, and showing support can mean a lot to someone else. When you cheer on others, you build a connection that strengthens the group dynamic. Providing suggestions or tips you have found useful can help others feel more confident in their practice. This supportive atmosphere can lead to friendships and a sense of belonging, which is essential for many people.

Lastly, it might be helpful to set personal goals within this online framework. Whether you want to improve your flexibility, strength, or overall fitness, having clear objectives will guide your involvement in the community. You might set a goal to practice three times a week or to try a new move each week. These small, achievable goals can keep your Pilates journey fresh and exciting. Writing down these goals can also serve as a reminder for you to stay focused and engaged.

Joining online platforms and social media groups dedicated to Pilates is a practical way to integrate this form of exercise into your routine. By being active in these communities, you can find support, share experiences, and stay motivated. The convenience of online platforms allows for flexibility while also connecting you with fellow Pilates enthusiasts from all walks of life. Embrace this digital space, participate, and enjoy the progress you can make.

Community Centers and Senior Centers

Community centers play a vital role in promoting wellness and fitness among different age groups, including seniors. These spaces are designed to be inclusive, allowing people from various backgrounds to come together. One of the key offerings at these centers is physical activity programs, such as Wall Pilates. These programs are not just about staying fit; they are also a way to create strong bonds between local residents. By joining in on group exercise classes, seniors can find companionship while taking part in activities that promote their health.

Finding the right community center or senior center is the first step towards engaging in these positive experiences. Start by doing some research on the programs available at your nearest facilities. You might be surprised at the range of options. Many centers offer fitness classes tailored specifically for seniors. These classes tend to focus on low-impact exercises, making them accessible for individuals who may have limitations due to age or health conditions. For instance, exercises that emphasize balance and core strength are particularly beneficial. They help in preventing falls, which is an important concern for older adults.

When you arrive at a community or senior center, you might find that the classes are often smaller in size. This is a deliberate choice that helps create a more personalized environment. With fewer participants, instructors can provide more attention to each individual. This one-on-one guidance can make a significant difference. It allows seniors to feel more comfortable as they try out new movements and exercises. The welcoming atmosphere fosters a sense of belonging; everyone can enjoy the benefits of exercise together.

Engagement in these local programs goes beyond just enhancing physical health. It also contributes positively to one's mental well-being. When seniors participate in group activities, they often feel less isolated. Sharing workouts with others builds a sense of community. This can be especially comforting for those who may live alone or have limited social interactions outside of their homes. Having a regular schedule to meet and exercise with others can create meaningful relationships. These connections can lead to friendships that extend beyond the fitness classes.

Taking part in classes is not only about the activity itself; it teaches participants how to care for their bodies effectively. In these sessions, seniors learn about different postures and movements. For example, Wall Pilates provides a unique way to engage with the workout. Participants can use the wall for support, making it easier to maintain balance while exercising. With each class, individuals become more aware of their body movements. This awareness can help in daily activities, allowing them to move more freely and confidently.

Engaging in these classes regularly can reinforce healthy habits. It encourages seniors to view fitness as a fun part of their life rather than a chore. When the exercises feel enjoyable and supportive, individuals are more likely to stick with them. Community centers often schedule a variety of classes throughout the week, giving participants the flexibility to find times that work best for their own schedules. They can explore different types of exercises, so they do not feel like they are doing the same thing every day.

Community centers frequently offer additional programs and resources for seniors. They may provide seminars on health topics, nutrition workshops, or social events that promote engagement. Attending these events is a valuable way to gain knowledge while also meeting new people. This combination of fitness and education creates a well-rounded experience for participants, making it easier for them to stay informed and active in their lives.

Finding a supportive environment can be motivating for seniors. When surrounded by peers who share similar goals, it's easier to stay committed to personal health. For example, after attending several classes together, it is common for participants to encourage one another. They might turn into workout buddies or even good friends, meeting outside of class for walks or coffee. This kind of support is invaluable. It enhances their fitness journey, making it a shared experience that adds joy to their daily lives.

For anyone interested in getting involved, visiting a community or senior center is a great next step. Take a tour of the facilities and ask about the programs available. Showing up is the best way to understand how these centers operate and what they offer. You can talk to instructors and current participants to gauge the atmosphere. Most importantly, this gives you a chance to see if you feel comfortable in the environment. A welcoming center will encourage you to join classes and participate regularly.

Do not hesitate to dive into new experiences. Each class is an opportunity to learn something new about your body and explore your physical abilities. The growth occurs not only in terms of fitness but also in building confidence and resilience. Every step taken within the support of a community center leads to a stronger and more connected individual. Engaging with others during these activities creates a cohesive network that can enhance both personal health and overall community spirit.

Participating in Pilates Forums and Websites

Engaging in Pilates forums and websites offers a wonderful opportunity to deepen your connection with the Pilates community. These platforms serve as gathering spots where individuals who share a passion for Pilates can come together. There are many different forums available, and each one provides an avenue for members to share their experiences, tips, and insights. This kind of interaction can greatly enhance your sense of belonging and help you feel more connected to others who share similar interests.

One of the most fulfilling aspects of participating in these online spaces is the chance to discuss various challenges that come with practicing Pilates. Everyone has obstacles, whether they are related to mastering a particular pose or maintaining motivation during training sessions. In forums, members often share their personal journeys, which can be incredibly inspiring. For example, if someone has struggled with a specific exercise, they might share techniques that worked for them or how they overcame their difficulties. This exchange can provide you with valuable strategies to apply to your own practice.

If you are considering diving into the world of Pilates forums, the first step is to identify reputable platforms. One of the most popular options is Reddit's Pilates community, where users can post questions, share their routines, and comment on others' experiences. Additionally, specialized websites like Pilates Anytime offer forums that allow practitioners to connect on a more focused level. These platforms are designed for those committed to Pilates, ensuring that discussions remain relevant and beneficial.

Once you select a forum that meets your needs, the next step is to create an account. Make sure to take the time to introduce yourself. Share your goals —whether you're a beginner looking to improve your flexibility or an experienced practitioner aiming to deepen your practice. This introduction is crucial because it sets the tone for your engagement with the community. It shows that you are willing to participate actively and opens the door for others to reach out and connect with you.

After you have made your introduction, it is essential to be proactive. Instead of simply lurking in the background, dive into discussions and respond to other members' posts. For instance, if someone shares a workout routine they enjoy, you can reply with your thoughts. Did you try it out? How did it work for you? Providing your input not only helps others but also fosters a sense of community. It builds relationships and encourages others to engage with you as well.

One of the great things about these forums is that they often include threads dedicated to asking for advice on specific exercises or routines. If you find yourself stuck on a particular move, don't hesitate to ask for help. Describe the challenges you are facing clearly and ask for tips. Chances are, someone else has experienced the same issue and can provide guidance based on their experiences. Sharing these struggles can lead to insightful conversations and support from the community.

Celebrating achievements is another beautiful aspect of engaging in Pilates forums. When you or another member reaches a personal milestone—be it mastering a challenging pose, completing a certain number of classes, or improving flexibility—share it! Recognition fosters an encouraging environment. Members appreciate these moments, and you may find that your simple post about a small victory can inspire someone else on their journey.

The relationships built through these forums can extend beyond just the virtual space. Many members may form friendships that lead to real-life meetups or group workouts. Connecting with others locally can offer additional motivation and a sense of accountability. When you have workout buddies, you're more likely to stay committed to your goals, as you'll want to show up for each other.

If you feel overwhelmed by the volume of information available, start by taking small steps. Read several posts each day to familiarize yourself with the community's dynamic and the topics that frequently arise. Keep a notebook for any valuable tips you come across. These notes will serve as a personalized compilation of ideas you can refer back to as you progress in your Pilates journey.

As you become more comfortable within the forum, explore other resources the platform may offer. These might include video tutorials, workout plans, or expert advice columns. Many forums collaborate with instructors and experienced practitioners who share their knowledge on various topics. Engaging with these resources can enhance your understanding of Pilates and improve your practice.

Always remember to be respectful and supportive when engaging with others. The atmosphere in these forums should remain positive and encouraging. If disagreements arise, approach them with kindness and a willingness to learn from differing opinions. Maintaining this respectful approach will contribute to a supportive community where everyone can thrive.

Joining Pilates forums and websites is an excellent way to strengthen your belonging to the

Pilates community. By exchanging experiences and tips, engaging in discussions, and supporting each other, members can create a network that transcends geographical boundaries. Each engagement can enrich your practice and help you build lasting relationships with fellow Pilates enthusiasts.

Sharing Experiences and Progress

Communicating one's fitness journey can significantly enhance motivation and foster connections within a community. When individuals share their progress and challenges, it creates a sense of accountability and encourages others to engage in similar positive behaviors.

Keeping a fitness journal is an effective way to document progress and boost self-confidence by recognizing growth over time. A journal allows individuals to reflect on their daily activities, note improvements, and identify areas that may need more attention. This process fosters a sense of accomplishment as the small victories become apparent. For seniors maintaining functional strength or beginners starting their Pilates journey, seeing tangible evidence of progress can be particularly motivating. Journaling also provides a structured space for setting goals and celebrating milestones, which are critical components of long-term success. Reflecting on past entries can serve as an inspiration during challenging times, reminding individuals of the progress they have made and the obstacles they have already overcome.

Posting achievements on social media invites encouragement from family and friends, creating accountability. By sharing accomplishments, whether it's mastering a new exercise or reaching a fitness goal, individuals can receive support and applause from their network. This public acknowledgment can greatly enhance motivation, making one feel part of a larger supportive community. Moreover, social media platforms enable interactions with others who are on similar fitness journeys, providing a sense of camaraderie and shared purpose. It's important, however, to approach this with balance; while sharing successes can be uplifting, it's equally valuable to post about challenges and setbacks to present a realistic picture of the journey. This honesty can foster deeper connections as others may relate to these experiences and offer valuable advice or empathy (The Importance of Accountability in Achieving Your Goals, 2023).

Engaging in fitness challenges provides opportunities to track progress publicly and build camaraderie. Challenges, whether organized through gyms, community groups, or online platforms, create a sense of friendly competition and collective effort.

Participants often find themselves pushing harder and staying committed when they know others are tracking their progress. For example, a month-long wall Pilates challenge can motivate participants to practice consistently, share their progress, and cheer each other on. These challenges not only enhance individual accountability but also build a sense of community among participants. The shared experience of working towards a common goal can create bonds and foster a supportive environment where members uplift each other. Participating in such challenges can introduce individuals to new exercises and techniques, broadening their fitness repertoire and keeping their routine interesting and dynamic.

Organizing feedback sessions fosters dialogue, refines personal practices, and enhances classroom environments. Regular feedback sessions, whether formal or informal, allow participants to discuss their experiences, share tips, and provide constructive feedback to each other. In a classroom setting, such sessions can help instructors understand the needs and preferences of their students better, allowing them to tailor classes more effectively. For example, incorporating a brief discussion period at the end of a Pilates class where participants can talk about what worked well and what they found challenging can be incredibly beneficial. This interaction not only improves personal practices by highlighting areas for improvement but also strengthens the sense of community as participants engage in meaningful dialogue. Feedback sessions also encourage active participation, making individuals feel valued and heard, thereby increasing their commitment to the program.

Participating in Group Challenges and Events

Engaging with community events and challenges can significantly enhance the Wall Pilates experience by creating an environment of motivation and accountability while fostering stronger community bonds. This can be done through various means such as local Pilates competitions, charity events, seasonal or themed challenges, and workshops and retreats.

Local Pilates competitions or showcases are excellent ways to promote friendly competition and motivate diligent practice among participants. These events provide a platform for individuals to display their skills and progress, which can be incredibly inspiring for both participants and spectators. For seniors who may be new to competitive environments, these competitions can be adjusted to cater to different skill levels, ensuring that everyone has the opportunity to participate. Beginners often find such settings encouraging, as they get to see firsthand the potential results of consistent practice. It's beneficial to join or organize events where there's a clear structure and support system, ensuring participants feel comfortable and motivated. Setting up a leaderboard or awarding small prizes can also add an element of fun and excitement, keeping participants engaged and driven to improve.

Charity Pilates events connect individuals with causes, adding meaning and unity to their practice. By aligning fitness goals with charitable activities, participants find greater purpose in their routines. For instance, organizing a Wall Pilates marathon where donations are collected based on the number of hours or specific exercises completed can galvanize participants to push their limits. Seniors might particularly enjoy this, as it combines physical activity with a cause they care about deeply. For beginners, the awareness that their efforts contribute to something larger than themselves can serve as a powerful motivator. When planning a charity event, it is essential to choose a cause that resonates with the majority of participants, ensuring higher engagement and enthusiasm. Collaborating with local businesses for sponsorships or partnerships can further expand the reach and impact of the event, promoting a sense of community involvement and support.

Seasonal or themed challenges are another excellent method to rekindle enthusiasm and prompt creative approaches to routine design. These challenges can range from a winter flexibility series to a summer strength challenge, each designed to keep the practice fresh and exciting. Seasonal themes can make the practice feel more relevant and engaging. For example, a "Spring Renewal" Wall Pilates challenge might focus on rejuvenating exercises that emphasize flexibility and fresh starts, appealing to seniors looking to improve their mobility and beginners seeking to establish a steady fitness routine. Themed challenges can also incorporate elements of fun, like costume days or special playlists, making the sessions enjoyable and something to look forward to. Setting up group challenges where progress can be monitored collectively helps build camaraderie and keeps participants motivated to stay on track.

Workshops and retreats offer immersive experiences that introduce new techniques and foster deep connections with like-minded individuals. Participating in a weekend retreat focused on advanced Wall Pilates techniques or attending a workshop led by expert instructors can provide invaluable learning opportunities. These events often delve deeper into the philosophy and finer points of Pilates practice, offering insights that regular classes might not cover. For seniors, workshops tailored towards gentle, yet effective movements can help address specific health concerns like joint pain or balance issues. Beginners, on the other hand, can benefit from foundational workshops that build their confidence and understanding of basic principles. Organizing or joining a retreat can also serve as a mini-vacation, combining relaxation with the opportunity to fully immerse oneself in the practice. It's crucial to ensure that these events are well-structured and inclusive, providing modifications for varying levels of ability and ensuring that all participants feel supported and challenged appropriately.

The social aspect of these events cannot be overstated. Building relationships with fellow practitioners through shared experiences creates a network of support that extends beyond the practice itself. Whether it's through exchanging tips on achieving difficult poses, sharing personal progress stories, or simply enjoying the company of others with similar interests, these interactions bolster a sense of belonging and community. For seniors, participating in a supportive and understanding community can alleviate feelings of isolation and provide a sense of purpose. For beginners, knowing that there's a community cheering them on can boost their confidence and motivation to stick with their fitness journey.

Reflecting on Our Journey

Engaging with communities, whether local or online, is essential for enhancing motivation and accountability in Wall Pilates practice. Throughout this chapter, we have explored various avenues to find supportive groups, such as local classes, community centers, and online platforms. These environments offer opportunities for social interaction, real-time feedback from instructors, and the exchange of valuable insights among practitioners. By actively participating in these communities, individuals can build strong networks that provide encouragement, advice, and a sense of belonging, making their Pilates practice more enriching and consistent.

Sharing personal experiences and progress within these communities further amplifies the benefits. Keeping a fitness journal or posting achievements on social media can boost self-confidence and invite supportive feedback from peers. Additionally, engaging in group challenges, competitions, and charity events fosters a sense of collective effort and friendly competition, which drives participants to stay committed. The integration of regular feedback sessions also enhances personal practices by encouraging open dialogue and mutual support. By embracing the resources and connections available within these communities, both seniors and beginners can achieve their fitness goals more effectively, enjoying a well-rounded and fulfilling Wall Pilates journey.

Conclusion

As we reach the end of this guide, it's essential to reflect on the key principles that have defined our journey together. Wall Pilates is more than just a series of exercises; it's about embracing an approach to movement that honors your unique body and circumstances. Whether you are a senior looking to maintain functional strength or a beginner venturing into the world of fitness, the principles we've explored can be tailored to suit your needs.

Throughout this book, we've delved into the fundamental aspects of Wall Pilates—posture, control, and breath. Each element plays a critical role in ensuring that your practice is safe, effective, and enjoyable. For seniors, this means adjusting movements to respect your body's limits, allowing for modifications that ensure safety while still providing a challenge. For beginners, it involves learning to move with intention, building a solid foundation that will support more complex exercises as you progress.

Understanding your body is paramount. It's about recognizing where you are today and working within those boundaries to foster growth. This awareness is a cornerstone of Wall Pilates, enabling you to make informed choices about each movement and modification. During our journey, we've emphasized how vital it is to listen to your body's signals—respecting its current capabilities while gently encouraging it towards greater strength and flexibility.

Wall Pilates offers a spectrum of holistic benefits that extend beyond physical fitness. Embracing this practice can significantly enhance not only your physical health but also your mental well-being. The interconnected nature of mind and body means that each stretch and movement contributes to a broader sense of balance and tranquility. Imagine initiating your day with gentle Wall Pilates exercises, paving the way for a calm and centered mindset that carries through your daily activities.

Physical benefits of Wall Pilates include improved strength, better balance, and enhanced flexibility. These aspects are crucial, particularly for seniors aiming to maintain independence and prevent injuries. For younger fitness enthusiasts, these benefits translate into a solid foundation upon which to build more rigorous activities, reducing the risk of injury and improving overall performance.

Mentally, practicing Wall Pilates can serve as a form of moving meditation. The focused concentration required helps quiet the mind, reduce stress, and promote a sense of inner peace. Incorporating mindful breathing techniques within your practice deepens this meditative aspect, fostering a calming environment that supports mental clarity and emotional stability.

Consistency is key to reaping the benefits of Wall Pilates. Establishing a regular practice routine ensures that the positive effects accumulate over time, gradually transforming your strength, flexibility, and balance. It's important to view this commitment not as a temporary endeavor but as a lifelong investment in your health and vitality. By dedicating just a few minutes each day to Wall Pilates, you lay the groundwork for sustained well-being.

As life evolves, so should your practice. Adaptability is integral to maintaining engagement and motivation. Seniors may find that their needs change over time, requiring adjustments to their routine to accommodate shifts in strength and mobility. Beginners will experience a natural progression, finding joy in mastering new exercises and challenges. This evolution keeps the practice fresh and exciting, continually offering new avenues for growth and improvement.

Engaging with a community can profoundly enrich your Wall Pilates journey. Whether you're connecting online or joining local classes, sharing experiences, challenges, and victories with like-minded individuals fosters a sense of belonging and motivation. For seniors, this connection can provide much-needed support and encouragement, making the practice more enjoyable and sustainable. For younger practitioners, being part of a community can spark inspiration, introduce new techniques, and create a network of accountability.

Communities offer a platform where stories are shared, advice is given, and achievements are celebrated. They serve as a reminder that you're not alone on this path. Engaging with others who share your passion for Wall Pilates can propel you forward, offering camaraderie and a collective drive to pursue wellness goals. These interactions can transform a solitary practice into a shared adventure, enriching your experience and broadening your horizons.

This journey doesn't end here. This book has provided you with tools, insights, and inspiration to carry forward. As you continue practicing Wall Pilates, remember that every movement counts, contributing to a healthier, more balanced life. The knowledge and skills you've acquired are stepping stones, each one building upon the last, forging a path towards enduring strength, flexibility, and peace.

In committing to Wall Pilates, you're nurturing a relationship with movement that adapts and grows with you, supporting you at every stage of life. For seniors, it's a pathway to maintaining independence, vitality, and joy in everyday activities. For younger beginners, it represents the beginning of a fitness journey characterized by confidence, strength, and a profound understanding of your body.

As you move forward, embrace each challenge with determination and each success with gratitude. Your dedication to Wall Pilates is a testament to your commitment to living a vibrant, healthy, and fulfilling life. Remember to celebrate your progress, no matter how small, and take pride in the resilience and strength you cultivate along the way.

Thank you for allowing me to be a part of your Wall Pilates journey. May this practice bring you strength, serenity, and a deeper connection to the wonderful capabilities of your body. Here's to a lifetime of health, happiness, and harmony through Wall Pilates.

References

A guide to basic stretches . (2023, August 30). Mayo Clinic. www.mayoclinic.org/healthy-lifestyle/fitness/in-depth/stretching/art-20546848

@anniepilatespt on TikTok - Make Your Day . (2024). Tiktok.com. www.tiktok.com/@anniepilatespt/video/7374648031616060714

Archer Pilates. (2018, June 15). *Archer Pilates* . archerpilates.com/therapeutic-pilates-pilates-exercises-lower-back-pain/

Barnes, M. (2023, November 13). *What Exactly Is Wall Pilates? Plus 5 Wall Pilates Exercises to Try at Home* . YouAligned. youaligned.com/fitness/what-is-wall-pilates/

Better Health Channel. (2012). *Osteoporosis and exercise* . Vic.gov.au. www.betterhealth.vic.gov.au/health/ConditionsAndTreatments/osteoporosis-and-exercise

Breitowich, A. (2024, April 24). *This At-Home Wall Pilates Workout Is Perfect For Beginners* . Women's Health. www.womenshealthmag.com/fitness/a46650229/wall-pilates/

Burgess, L. (2019, March 8). *Top 10 shoulder stretches for pain and tightness* .

Www.medicalnewstoday.com.
www.medicalnewstoday.com/articles/324647

Cleveland Clinic. (2023, March 10). *Pilates 101: What It Is and Its Health Benefits* . Cleveland Clinic. health.clevelandclinic.org/everything-you-want-to-know-about-pilates

Cleveland Clinic. (2021, June 2). *Worried About Falling? Try These Exercises to Improve Your Balance* . Cleveland Clinic; Cleveland Clinic. health.clevelandclinic.org/worried-about-falling-try-these-exercises-to-improve-your-balance

Core Stabilization Program . (n.d.). Peak Sport & Spine. peaksportspine.com/core-stabilization-program/

Creating Your Home Pilates Studio: Equipment Essentials and Layout Ideas - Go Align Pilates . (2024, March 2). Go Align Pilates. goalignpilates.com/creating-your-home-pilates-studio-equipment-essentials-and-layout-ideas/

Cronkleton, E. (2019, March 22). *Balance exercises: 13 Moves with Instructions* . Healthline. www.healthline.com/health/exercises-for-balance

Curley, E. (2019, November 29). *5 Great Fitness Challenge Ideas for Charity* . Glofox. www.glofox.com/blog/fitness-challenges-for-charity/

de Mille, P. (2022, June 9). 6 Simple Ways to Increase Your Flexibility. Hospital for Special Surgery. www.hss.edu/article_how-to-increase-flexibility.asp

Downey, J. (2024, February 20). *I tried a 15-minute wall Pilates workout — here are my honest thoughts* . Tom's Guide; Tom's Guide. www.tomsguide.com/wellness/fitness/i-tried-a-15-minute-wall-pilates-workout-here-are-my-honest-thoughts

Ellwand, O. (2023, May 17). *What is Pilates? How to Get Started With Pilates* . merrithew. www.merrithew.com/blog/post/2023-05-17/what-is-pilates-everything-you-need-to-know-about-pilates

Evergreen. (2023, July). *This Pilates wall workout is the summer's top workout.* Evergreen Rehab and Wellness. evergreenclinic.ca/this-pilates-wall-workout-is-the-summers-top-workout/

Exercising With Chronic Conditions . (n.d.). National Institute on Aging. www.nia.nih.gov/health/exercise-and-physical-activity/exercising-chronic-conditions

FasterCapital. (n.d.). *Community challenges or contests: Fitness challenges: Sweat and success: The growing trend of fitness challenges* . Retrieved from fastercapital.com/content/Community-challenges-or-contests--Fitness-Challenges--Sweat-and-Success--The-Growing-Trend-of-Fitness-Challenges.html

Fitness Social Media Content Ideas [+ AI Social Post Generator] . (2024, August 19). StoryLab.ai. storylab.ai/examples/fitness-social-media-content-ideas/

Hammond, B. (2024). *Wall Pilates exercises: What are the benefits? GoodRx Health* . www.goodrx.com/well-being/movement-exercise/wall-pilates-exercises

Hardy, L. (2024, January 3). *Age-Specific Wall Pilates Routines* . wall pilates. wallpilates.com/age-specific-wall-pilates-routines/

Hardy, L. (2024, April 11). *Building Self-Esteem Through Wall Pilates* . wall pilates. wallpilates.com/building-self-esteem-through-wall-pilates/

Hardy, L. (2024, January 29). *Pilates for Post-Operative Recovery* . wall pilates. wallpilates.com/pilates-for-post-operative-recovery/

Hardy, L. (2024, April 2). *The Role of Community in Wall Pilates Practice* . wall pilates. wallpilates.com/the-role-of-community-in-wall-pilates-practice/

Hardy, L. (2024, April 10). *Stress Reduction with Wall Pilates.* wall pilates. wallpilates.com/stress-reduction-with-wall-pilates/

Hardy, L. (2024, January 11). *Upper Body Workouts with Wall Pilates.* wall pilates. wallpilates.com/upper-body-workouts-with-wall-pilates/

Hardy, L. (2024, February 17). *Wall Pilates and Cardiovascular Training.* wall pilates. wallpilates.com/wall-pilates-and-cardiovascular-training/

Hardy, L. (2024, January 21). *Wall Pilates and Mind-Body Connection Exercises* . wall pilates.

wallpilates.com/wall-pilates-and-mind-body-connection-exercises/

Hardy, L. (2024, January 15). *Wall Pilates Breathing Techniques* . wall pilates. wallpilates.com/wall-pilates-breathing-techniques/

Hardy, L. (2023, July 14). *Wall Pilates Exercises For Seniors*. wall pilates. wallpilates.com/wall-pilates-exercises-for-seniors/

Hardy, L. (2024, January 14). *Wall Pilates for Balance and Stability* . wall pilates. wallpilates.com/wall-pilates-for-balance-and-stability/

Hardy, L. (2024, March 31). *Wall Pilates for Mindfulness and Focus.* wall pilates. wallpilates.com/wall-pilates-for-mindfulness-and-focus/

Hardy, L. (2024, January 24). *Wall Pilates for Seniors: Improving Balance* . wall pilates. wallpilates.com/wall-pilates-for-seniors-improving-balance/

Hardy, L. (2024, January 25). *Wall Pilates Workouts for Small Spaces.* wall pilates. wallpilates.com/wall-pilates-workouts-for-small-spaces/

Isacowitz, R. & Clippinger, K. (2020). *Pilates Anatomy* . (2nd Edition). Human Kinetics.

Kloubec, J. (2011). *Pilates: how does it work and who needs it?* Muscles, Ligaments and Tendons

Journal; CIC Edizioni Internazionali. www.ncbi.nlm.nih.gov/pmc/articles/PMC3666467/

Lim, E.-J., & Hyun, E.-J. (2021, April 6). *The Impacts of Pilates and Yoga on Health-Promoting Behaviors and Subjective Health Status* . International Journal of Environmental Research and Public Health. doi.org/10.3390/ijerph18073802

Lindberg, S. (2020, January 10). *Shoulder Mobility Exercises and Stretches with Pictures* . Healthline. www.healthline.com/health/shoulder-mobility-exercises

Loren, K. (2023, November 17). *I Tried BetterMe Wall Pilates for 14 Days: Here's What Happened* . Women's Health. www.womenshealthmag.com/fitness/a45700748/i-tried-betterme-wall-pilates-for-14-days-heres-what-happened/

Maheshwari, S. (2024, June 27). *How to Make Your Pilates Program Stand Out* . Smart Health Clubs. smarthealthclubs.com/blog/how-to-make-your-pilates-program-stand-out/

Martin, S. (2020, August 19). *8 effective Pilates back exercises at home | Pilates for back pain (upper and lower)* . Complete Pilates. complete-pilates.co.uk/back-exercises-at-home/

Merrithew. (n.d.). *STOTT PILATES Basic Principles: Breathing* . merrithew. www.merrithew.com/stott-pilates/warmup/en/principles/breathing

Mulcahy, J . (2020, June 2). *6 Exercises to Promote Balance That You Can Do at Home* . Choose PT. www.choosept.com/health-tips/6-exercises-promote-balance-home

One Medical. (2021, May 25). *9 Stretching Exercises for Seniors*. onemedical. www.onemedical.com/blog/exercise-fitness/stretching-exercises-for-seniors/

Oravisto, J. (2023, November 23). *10 Best Home Pilates Equipment (The Ultimate Beginner Guide)* . Blog | BAY STUDIOS. b log.bay-studios.com/best-home-pilates-equipment/

Page, D. (2023, September 12). *People are raving about wall Pilates for fast results. Find out why it's so effective* . TODAY. www.today.com/health/diet-fitness/wall-pilates-exercises-rcna103846

Pedersen, H., Fimland, M. S., Schoenfeld, B. J., Iversen, V. M., Cumming, K. T., Jensen, S., Saeterbakken, A. H., & Andersen, V. (2022, May 14). *A randomized trial on the efficacy of split-body versus full-body resistance training in non-resistance trained women* . BMC Sports Science, Medicine and Rehabilitation. doi.org/10.1186/s13102-022-00481-7

Read, T. (2024, April 17). *10 Best Low-Impact Exercises for Seniors* . AOL. www.aol.com/10-best-low-impact-exercises-100006105.html

7 Simple Stretches for Older Adults . (2019, September 18). SilverSneakers.

www.silversneakers.com/blog/stretching-for-seniors-7-simple-moves-for-the-not-so-flexible/

Shelly, I. (2024, April 30). *Pilates Equipment Essentials: Building the Perfect Home Studio for Total Body Conditioning* . Pilates Reformers Plus. pilatesreformersplus.com/blogs/news/pilates-equipment-essentials-building-the-perfect-home-studio-for-total-body-conditioning

Sparks, J. (2024, April 15). *Top 10 Wall Pilates Apps of 2024* . wall pilates. wallpilates.com/top-10-wall-pilates-apps-of-2024/

Spraul, T. (2024, January 5). *Gym Design Guide (Pictures, Ideas, and Tips).* Exercise.com www.exercise.com/grow/gym-design-guide/

Spraul, T. (2023, May 29). *What features should a fitness app have?* Exercise.com www.exercise.com/grow/what-features-should-a-fitness-app-have/

Stogdon, M. (2024, July 4). *Wall Pilates Workout for Core Strengthening* . PROMiXX. www.promixx.com/en-gb/blogs/academy/wall-pilates-workout

The Importance Of Accountability In Achieving Your Goals . (2023, July 28). Theaspireclub. theaspireclub.com/the-importance-of-accountability-in-achieving-your-goals/

12 Scientifically Proven Benefits of Pilates for Your Peace of Mind . (2013, September 25). Pilates Bridge. pilatesbridge.com/12-scientifically-proven-benefits-of-pilates-for-your-peace-of-mind/

Valcarce-Torrente, M., Javaloyes, V., Gallardo, L., García-Fernández, J., & Planas-Anzano, A. (2021, January 1). *Influence of Fitness Apps on Sports Habits, Satisfaction, and Intentions to Stay in Fitness Center Users: An Experimental Study* . International Journal of Environmental Research and Public Health. doi.org/10.3390/ijerph181910393

Ventana by Buckner. (2023, May 23). *Wall Pilates for Seniors* . Ventana by Buckner. www.ventanabybuckner.com/blog/wall-pilates-for-seniors/

Walters, J. (2021, September 22). *7 Expert Tips For Improving Flexibility* . Forbes Health. www.forbes.com/health/fitness/how-to-improve-flexibility/

Ward, S. (2022, February 15). *How to Engage Your Core: Steps, Muscles Worked, and More* . Healthline. www.healthline.com/nutrition/how-to-engage-your-core

Yasinski, E. (2024, January 12). *A Pilates Routine You Can Do Anywhere in Under 10 Minutes* . The New York Times. www.nytimes.com/2024/01/12/well/move/pilates-workout-at-home.html

Yetman, D. (2020, May 28). *Muscle Groups to Work Out Together: How to Create a Plan* . Healthline.

www.healthline.com/health/exercise-fitness/muscle-groups-to-workout-together